KV-699-429

Contents

Preface		*page* vii
Installation Instructions		viii
Note on QBase		ix
Abbreviations		x
Exam 1	Questions	1
Exam 1	Answers	15
Exam 2	Questions	26
Exam 2	Answers	39
Exam 3	Questions	50
Exam 3	Answers	63
Exam 4	Questions	74
Exam 4	Answers	87
Exam 5	Questions	98
Exam 5	Answers	111
Exam 1	Supplementary Questions	122
Exam 1	Supplementary Answers	124
Exam 2	Supplementary Questions	125
Exam 2	Supplementary Answers	127
Exam 3	Supplementary Questions	128
Exam 3	Supplementary Answers	130
Exam 4	Supplementary Questions	131
Exam 4	Supplementary Answers	133
Exam 5	Supplementary Questions	134
Exam 5	Supplementary Answers	136

QBASE PAEDIATRICS 2
MCQS FOR THE PART A DCH

QBASE PAEDIATRICS 2
MCQS FOR THE PART A DCH

Rachel U. Sidwell
MRCP, MRCPH, DFFP, DA

Mike Thomson
FRCP, FRCPH, DCH, MD

With contributions from James S. A. Green,
FRCS, LLM, Whipps Cross Hospital

QBase developed and edited by
Edward Hammond

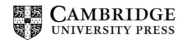

CAMBRIDGE UNIVERSITY PRESS
Cambridge, New York, Melbourne, Madrid, Cape Town, Singapore, São Paulo, Delhi

Cambridge University Press
The Edinburgh Building, Cambridge CB2 8RU, UK

Published in the United States of America by Cambridge University Press, New York

www.cambridge.org
Information on this title: www.cambridge.org/9780521698368

© Cambridge University Press 2008

First published 2008

Printed in the United Kingdom at the University Press, Cambridge

A catalogue record for this publication is available from the British Library

Library of Congress Cataloguing in Publication Data

Sidwell, Rachel U.
QBase paediatrics 2 : MCQs for the Part A DCH / Rachel U. Sidwell, Mike Thomson; with
contributions from James S. A. Green; QBase developed and edited by Edward Hammond.
p. ; cm.
Includes bibliographical references and index.
ISBN 978-0-521-69836-8 (pbk.)
1. Pediatrics–Examinations, questions, etc.   I. Thomson, Mike (Mike Andrew)
II. Green, James S. A.   III. Hammond, Edward.   IV. Title.
[DNLM: 1. Pediatrics.   2. Examination Questions.   WS 18.2 S596q 2008]
RJ48.2.S32 2008
618.9200076–dc22   2008006279

ISBN 978-0-521-69836-8 paperback

Preface

The questions in this book focus on areas of child health relevant to general paediatrics as encountered by primary care physicians as well as paediatricians. This book is an aid for both those taking the MRCPCH and those taking the DCH.

The questions in this book are multiple true–false questions (MCQs), also available on the accompanying CD-ROM, allowing practice in this component of the exam (which is the key to passing MCQs) and also making this process a little more fun. The CD-ROM allows the questions to be randomly 'scrambled', and for methodical learning, questions on a particular subject can also be selected separately and a single topic covered in detail. In addition, there are a few example questions of the 'best of five' and 'extended match' type included at the end of the book to allow the reader to get a feel for the structure of these other question types.

The MRCPCH Part 1 exam consists of Paper One A and Paper One B. Paper One A forms part of the MRCPCH Part 1 examination, and also the written examination for the Diploma in Child Health (DCH). The exam format will be changing again (and it is advisable to check the college website, www.rcpch.ac.uk/Examinations, for any further changes). Since January 2008, both paper 1A and paper 1B consist of 69 questions made up of the following:

- 25 Multiple true–false questions (MCQ)
- 35 Best of five questions (BOF)
- 9 Extended match questions (EMQ)

Remember to read each question carefully, and do not be caught out by simple phraseology. Look out for key phrases such as 'always' and 'never' both of which are unlikely to be true. Terms such as 'commonly', 'usually' and 'often' are unfortunately ambiguous and open to interpretation. And finally remember that even if you think you know nothing about a question, you must answer as intelligently as you can because your probability of being right is more than that of being wrong, simply because you are making an educated guess.

Have fun, and best of luck!

RUS
MT

Installation Instructions

QBASE PAEDIATRICS 2 ON CD-ROM MINIMUM
SYSTEM REQUIREMENTS

- An IBM compatible PC with a 80386 processor and 4 MB of RAM
- VGA monitor set up to display at least 256 colours
- CD-ROM drive
- Windows 95 or higher with Microsoft compatible mouse

NB: The display setting of your computer must be set to display 'SMALL FONTS' (see MS Windows manuals for further instructions on how to do this if necessary)

INSTALLATION INSTRUCTIONS

The program will install the appropriate files onto your hard drive. It requires the QBase CD-ROM to be in installed in the CD-ROM drive (usually drives D: or E:).

In order to run QBase, the CD must be in the drive

Print **Readme.txt** and **Helpfile.txt** on the CD-ROM for fuller instructions and user manual

WINDOWS 95, 98, 2000, XP

1. Insert the QBase CD-ROM into the drive
2. From the Start Menu, select the Run... option, type **D:\setup.exe** (where D: is the CD-ROM drive) and press OK or open the contents of the CD-ROM and double-click the **setup.exe** icon
3. Follow the 'Full – install all files' to accept the default directory for installation of QBase
4. Click 'Yes' to the prompt 'Do you want setup to create Program Manager groups?' If you have a previously installed version of QBase, click 'Yes' to the next prompt 'Should the new Program Manager groups replace existing duplicate groups?'
5. To run QBase, go to the Start Menu, then Programs, QBase and **QBase Exam.** From Windows Explorer, double-click the **QBase.exe** file in the QBase folder on your hard drive.

Note on QBase

Notes for users of *QBase Paediatrics 2* on CD-ROM

Please read carefully and print the HELPFILE on the QBase CD-ROM as it contains detailed information on the features and analysis functions of QBase.

QBase is an interactive MCQ examination program designed to help candidates improve their performance in MCQs. Please follow the installation instructions printed on the previous page. Once installed, the QBase program resides on your hard disk and reads the data from whatever QBase CD is in your CD drive. If you install QBase from this CD, it will update any previous version of the program. Owners of previous QBase titles will then have access to any new functions available on this new version of the program. All QBase CDs will work with the new program. To check for successful installation of the new program, check the Quick Start Menu screen: it should have 5 exam buttons.

QBase Paediatrics 2 contains 325 questions for the Part A DCH. The 'Autoset Exam' option on this CD will present you with an exam of 65 questions, utilizing any of the 325 questions on the CD. The 5 predefined exams on the CD are constructed in the same way, and are exactly the same as the 5 exams printed in this book. You can also generate your own customized exams using the 'Create your own exam' option. You can save completed exams and your responses to your hard disk, allowing you to review or resit the same paper at a later stage in your revision. Please refer to the helpfile on the CD for more information. To further enhance your revision, instead of selecting the 'Resit exam' option, we suggest that you try the 'Resit shuffled exam' option. The leaves within each question will then be randomly shuffled, removing your ability to remember the pattern of correct answers rather than the facts. The exam analysis functions of QBase will provide you with a detailed breakdown of your performance.

Abbreviations

ADH	antidiuretic hormone
ADHD	attention deficit hyperactivity disorder
ALL	acute lymphocytic leukaemia
ANA	antinuclear antibody
ASD	atrial septal defect
BCG	Bacille Calmette-Guérin
CHD	congenital heart disease
CNS	central nervous system
CT	computed tomography
CXR	chest X-ray
DNA	deoxyribonucleic acid
ECG	electrocardiogram
EEG	electro-encephalogram
FSH	follicle-stimulating hormone
GI tract	gastrointestinal tract
GOR	gastro-oesophageal reflux
G6PD	glucose-6 phosphate dehydrogenase
Hb	haemoglobin
HCG	human chorionic gonadotrophin
HHV-6	human herpes virus 6
HIV	human immunodeficiency virus
HSV	herpes simplex virus
5-HT	5-hydroxytryptamine
LH	luteinizing hormone
MMR	measles, mumps, rubella
MRI	magnetic resonance imaging
PCR	polymerase chain reaction
PPI	proton pump inhibitor
RNA	ribonucleic acid
RSV	respiratory syncytial virus
SIADH	syndrome of inappropriate antidiuretic hormone
SIDS	sudden infant death syndrome
SLE	systemic lupus erythematosus
TB	tuberculosis

UTI	urinary tract infection
VSD	ventricular septal defect
vWF	von Willebrand factor
VZIG	varicella zoster immunoglobulin

Q 1.   **Typical febrile convulsions**

    A. Occur between 3 months and 5 years
    B. Are seen in 10% of children
    C. Have a genetic predisposition
    D. May be focal
    E. Should always be managed with rectal diazepam

Q 2.   **The following are true of cerebral palsy**

    A. It can be difficult to diagnose during the first year of life
    B. It is commonly associated with faltering growth
    C. A low 5-minute Apgar score correlates well with development of cerebral palsy
    D. Seizures are most commonly seen in association with ataxic cerebral palsy
    E. Mental retardation is most commonly associated with dyskinetic cerebral palsy

Q 3.   **Regarding headaches**

    A. Recurrent tension headaches are experienced by around 1 in 10 children
    B. Recurrent headaches are a common symptom of non-organic illness in children
    C. They are more commonly seen in adolescents than in preschool children
    D. They are more frequent in boys
    E. They may be secondary to sinusitis

Q 4.   **Typical absence seizures**

    A. Are usually associated with developmental delay
    B. Last no longer than 1 minute
    C. Usually begin in school age children

D. Can be induced by hyperventilation

E. Usually continue in adult life

Q 5. A normal 6-month-old infant can

A. Transfer objects from one hand to the other

B. Release objects

C. Eat finger foods

D. Wave bye-bye

E. Sit well unaided

Q 6. A normally developing 1-year-old

A. Has a pincer grasp

B. Can pull to stand

C. May bottom-shuffle

D. Can do circular scribbles

E. Can feed with a spoon

Q 7. By 3 years of age, a normally developing child would be expected to

A. Kick

B. Jump

C. Stand on one leg

D. Hop

E. Ride a bicycle

Q 8. The following skills are correctly age-matched in a normally developing child

A. Hop on one leg by 3 years

B. Build a bridge with 3 cubes by 2 years

C. Say 2-word sentences by 18 months

D. Say Daddy non-specifically by 9 months

E. Name colours by 2 years

Q 9. The following primitive reflexes are present at 4 months

A. The palmar grasp

B. The plantar grasp

C. The Moro reflex

D. The asymmetric tonic neck reflex

E. The stepping reflex

Q 10. The following are true

A. Cerebral palsy is associated with motor delay

B. Autism is associated with a communication delay

C. A lack of stimulation can result in global delay

D. A child with an IQ of 20–50 has moderate learning disability

E. Cleft palate if untreated can cause a communication delay

Q 11. The following are prenatal screening tests

A. Chorionic villous sampling

B. Nuchal ultrasound scan

C. Amniocentesis

D. Fetal anomaly ultrasound scan

E. Percutaneous umbilical blood sampling

Q 12. The following conditions are diagnosable by fetal ultrasound at 20 weeks

A. Gastroschisis

B. Encephalocele

C. Cleft lip

D. Diaphragmatic hernia

E. Polycystic kidneys

Q 13. Down's syndrome babies

A. Have hypertonia at birth

B. Have hyperflexible joints

C. Have overlapping of the fifth finger over the fourth

D. Have a short tongue

E. Have small ears

Q 14. Turner syndrome infants

A. Have the karyotype 46,XO

B. May have congenital lymphoedema

C. Have a micropenis

D. Have microphthalmia

E. Have widely spaced nipples

Q 15. Regarding squints

A. The cover test is used to detect an alternating squint

B. Any squint present after 3 months of age should be referred to an ophthalmologist

C. Intermittent divergent squints can become constant with tiredness

D. A long-sighted child will have an accommodative convergent squint

E. Visual acuity must be assessed as part of squint assessment

Q 16. The following features would make one concerned that periorbital cellulitis had progressed to orbital cellulitis

A. Impaired colour vision

B. Proptosis

C. Fever

D. Normal acuity

E. Deafness

Q 17. Astigmatism

A. Can cause headaches

B. Can be corrected with glasses

C. Is a cause of amblyopia

D. Usually requires corrective surgery

E. Can manifest with the child holding books very close

Q 18. A child who has had a splenectomy

A. Will have a low platelet count

B. Is susceptible to infection with pneumococcus

C. Should have prophylactic penicillin for the first 2 months

D. Should have vaccination against diphtheria prior to splenectomy

E. Should have vaccination against meningococcus prior to splenectomy

Q 19. Iron deficiency anaemia

A. Is uncommon in infants

B. Is more likely to occur in premature infants

C. Is less common in formula-fed infants

D. Is associated with increased behavioural problems in toddlers

E. Is most commonly due to coeliac disease

Q 20. The commonest cause(s) of erythema multiforme in children is/are

A. Post-infection

B. Herpes simplex virus

C. Drugs

D. *Streptococcus* infection

E. Urticaria

Q 21. Port-wine stains

A. Are not usually apparent at birth

B. Are usually palpable

C. Are seen in about 5% of infants

D. May obscure vision if they involve the eyelid

E. Should be treated with the pulsed dye laser

Q 22. Regarding scabies infection in infants

A. It causes an asymptomatic papulo-vesicular rash

B. The rash typically affects the sides of the feet

C. The rash does not involve the scalp

D. The rash resolves within 1 week of treatment

E. Close contacts should be treated only if symptomatic

Q 23. Occult spinal dysraphism may present with the following midline lumbar skin features

A. Skin tags

B. Hypopigmentation

C. Lipoma

D. Port-wine stain

E. Hypertrichosis

Q 24. Phenylketonuria

A. Is a mucopolysaccharidosis

B. Causes cardiomyopathy

C. Causes developmental delay

D. Results from a deficiency in the enzyme to metabolize phenylalanine

E. Presents with an infant who is normal at birth

Q 25. In an infant with gastro-oesophageal reflux

A. Sudden infant death syndrome is a recognized sequela

B. Due to cow's milk sensitivity, the milk of choice is soya-based

C. An examination of a bag urine or MSU is not necessary

D. There is a 90–95% chance of complete resolution by 2 years of age

E. A reflux index (time below pH of 4) of 5% is considered to lie within the normal range

Q 26. The following can cause cirrhosis in childhood

A. Post stem cell transplant veno-occlusive disease

B. α-1-antitrypsin disease

C. Acute viral hepatitis

D. Autoimmune hepatitis

E. Biliary atresia with Kasai performed at 80 days of age

Q 27. Breast-fed infants

A. Have fewer episodes of otitis media than formula-fed infants

B. Have increased host defence proteins in the gastrointestinal tract

C. Have a lower incidence of respiratory infections than formula-fed infants

D. Have lower levels of secretory IgA than formula-fed infants

E. Have a higher incidence of gastrointestinal illness than formula-fed infants

Q 28. The following are features of an innocent childhood murmur

A. Changes with altered position of the child

B. Radiation to the neck

C. It becomes more pronounced with fever

D. There is never a diastolic component

E. The murmur is harsh

Q 29. In cardiac failure in an infant

A. It may present with chest infections
B. Hepatomegaly is generally present
C. The lungs often sound clear on auscultation
D. Feeding is usually normal
E. Peripheral oedema is present

Q 30. In an infant with suspected congenital heart disease the most useful initial investigation(s) would be

A. ECG
B. Chest X-ray (CXR)
C. Echocardiogram
D. Cardiac catheterization
E. Blood pressure analysis

Q 31. Urinary tract infection

A. Can present with sepsis in an infant
B. Is more common in boys than girls
C. Is associated with urinary tract abnormality in approximately 50% of cases
D. Is never asymptomatic in children
E. Is most commonly due to *Streptococcus* infection

Q 32. Nocturnal enuresis

A. Is seen in 10% of normal 5-year-olds
B. Is usually of organic cause
C. Requires neurological examination as routine
D. May be managed using anticholinergics
E. Is usually successfully resolved with psychological therapy in children over 5 years

Q 33. Perthes disease

A. Most commonly presents in adolescent boys
B. Is usually bilateral
C. May present with knee pain
D. Causes unequal leg length
E. Is not visible on plain X-ray

Q 34. Systemic onset juvenile idiopathic arthritis

A. Does not involve the joints
B. May mimic the symptoms of malignancy
C. Is a cause of hepatosplenomegaly
D. May cause pleuritis
E. Affects girls more than boys

Q 35. Kawasaki disease

A. Is a polyarteritis
B. Causes coronary artery aneurysms in up to 5% of untreated children
C. Causes a thrombocytopenia
D. Is managed with intravenous immunoglobulin if coronary artery aneurysms develop
E. Requires echocardiography only if there are cardiac signs or symptoms

Q 36. Congenital dislocation of the hip

A. Is associated with polyhydramnios
B. Should be screened for in all breech infants
C. Has an incidence of 1 in 10 000 births
D. Is more common in boys
E. May occur secondary to spina bifida

Q 37. The following may cause a painless limp in a child

A. A short limb
B. Osteomyelitis
C. Slipped upper femoral epiphysis
D. Irritable hip
E. Perthes disease

Q 38. The following hearing tests are appropriately age-matched

A. Performance testing – 1 year
B. Speech discrimination testing – 2–4 years
C. Distraction testing – 6 months
D. Pure tone audiometry – birth
E. Otoacoustic emissions – 9–24 months

Q 39. **Cystic fibrosis is the most likely diagnosis in a child with**

   A. Severe wheeze and failure to thrive
   B. Nasal polyps
   C. Recurrent chest infections and malabsorption
   D. Intussusception
   E. Right heart failure

Q 40. **Asthma**

   A. Is more common in boys
   B. Presents by the age of 3 years in 80% of cases
   C. Usually resolves by early adulthood
   D. Is associated with exercise-induced wheeze in 50% of cases
   E. Results in hypercapnoea in a mild attack

Q 41. **The following features in a 2.5-year-old child would indicate the possibility of autism**

   A. Developmental stasis
   B. Early language development
   C. Repetitive play
   D. Echolalia
   E. Late development of number recognition

Q 42. **The following are features of bulimia**

   A. Fear of becoming obese
   B. Laxative abuse
   C. Teeth enamel erosion
   D. Salivary gland enlargement
   E. Electrolyte abnormalities

Q 43. **Night terrors in infancy**

   A. Occur during REM sleep
   B. Are readily recalled on waking
   C. Tend to occur near to morning
   D. Are associated with sweating
   E. Last about half an hour

Q 44. **Amniocentesis can lead to prenatal detection of**

A. Microcephaly
B. Trisomy 18
C. Spina bifida cystica
D. Congenital infection
E. Trisomy 13

Q 45. **The following conditions can cause decreased maternal serum α-fetoprotein**

A. Multiple pregnancy
B. Open spina bifida
C. Fetomaternal haemorrhage
D. Trisomy 21
E. Polycystic kidney disease

Q 46. **The following are true of body temperature in a term newborn**

A. Shivering is important to maintain body heat
B. Sweating is used to regulate temperature
C. Brown fat is used to maintain body heat
D. Hypothermia may indicate sepsis
E. Ambient humidity will decrease evaporative losses

Q 47. **The following are true regarding sudden infant death syndrome**

A. It is most common during the neonatal period
B. Overheating is a risk factor
C. It is less common if the infant sleeps in the parents' bedroom
D. It is significantly more common in babies whose mothers smoked during pregnancy
E. The coroner is legally bound to hold an inquest

Q 48. **The following would be cause for concern in a 24-hour baby check**

A. A bulging anterior fontanelle
B. Erythema toxicum neonatorum
C. Cyanosis of the tongue
D. A red reflex
E. Peeling of the hands

Q 49. Regarding Vitamin K administration to newborns

    A. Is given to prevent thrombocytopenia of the newborn
    B. Promotes synthesis of clotting factor VIII
    C. Is less necessary in breast-fed infants
    D. Is necessary for the extrinsic coagulation pathway
    E. Is contraindicated if the mother has been taking phenytoin

Q 50. The following features would support a diagnosis of type 2 diabetes mellitus

    A. Normal weight
    B. Acanthosis nigricans
    C. Positive family history
    D. Ketonuria
    E. The presence of islet cell antibodies

Q 51. Hyperthyroidism during childhood may cause

    A. Delayed puberty
    B. Precocious puberty
    C. Hypercalcaemia
    D. Diarrhoea
    E. Cardiomegaly

Q 52. The following are suggestive of short stature due to constitutional delay

    A. Head circumference, height and weight all below the 3rd percentile
    B. Height delayed more than weight
    C. Bone age falling progressively further behind chronological age
    D. Sibling history of delayed development
    E. Bone age delayed by 5 years

Q 53. Gynaecomastia in a normal 15-year-old boy

    A. Usually resolves spontaneously within 3 months
    B. Is more common in overweight boys
    C. May involve only one breast if physiological
    D. Occurs to some degree in up to 25% of boys
    E. Often requires medical or surgical therapy

Q 54. Chloramphenicol may cause

    A. Nocturnal haemoglobinuria
    B. Peripheral neuritis
    C. Nephrotic syndrome
    D. Eosinophilia
    E. Red man syndrome

Q 55. Carbamazepine

    A. Is the first-line treatment of juvenile myoclonic epilepsy
    B. Commonly causes allergic rashes
    C. Is an enzyme inhibitor
    D. Is a sodium channel blocker
    E. May cause irreversible alopecia

Q 56. Kawasaki disease

    A. Is caused by HSV type 5 infection
    B. Is characterized by purulent conjunctivitis
    C. Classically is characterized by an irritable child
    D. Should be treated with aspirin
    E. Can be diagnosed after 48 hours of fever

Q 57. Mumps infection

    A. Is most common in the autumn
    B. Commonly involves solely the submandibular glands
    C. Is a rare cause of viral meningitis
    D. May cause transient hearing loss
    E. Is a cause of trismus

Q 58. Measles

    A. Has a 3-day incubation period
    B. Classically begins with a peripheral rash
    C. Koplik's spots develop on the gums just after the rash appears
    D. Commonly causes encephalitis
    E. Causes a lymphopenia

Q 59. Chicken pox

    A. Has a 10-day incubation period
    B. Is usually characterized with a prodromal illness in young children

C. Is commonly complicated by pneumonia in children

D. Is an RNA virus

E. Can cause congenital malformation if present in a pregnant mother

Q 60. Hand, foot and mouth disease

A. Is caused by a paramyxovirus infection

B. Is transmitted by droplet route

C. Is usually seen in school age children

D. Can cause an arthritis

E. Commonly features papules on the buttocks

Q 61. Whooping cough

A. Is caused by a paramyxovirus

B. Is spread by the faecal-oral route

C. May cause rectal prolapse

D. Is treated with ribavirin

E. Has a 3-day incubation period

Q 62. The following are contraindications to vaccination

A. A cold

B. Severe local reaction to previous dose

C. Acute febrile illness

D. Neonatal jaundice

E. Family history of convulsions

Q 63. The BCG

A. Is an inactivated virus

B. Should be given if the tuberculin test is positive

C. Can be given if the child has widespread impetigo

D. Should not be given to an HIV positive child

E. Should not be given to a child with leukaemia

Q 64. A child with HIV

A. Should not be given pertussis vaccination

B. May receive the intramuscular poliomyelitis vaccination

C. Should be given the BCG if the tuberculin test is negative

D. Can be given the Hib vaccine

E. Should not be given the MMR

Q 65. Diphtheria vaccination

A. Is contraindicated in a child on high dose steroids
B. Is given as a booster dose at 1 year
C. Should not be given to a child with slapped cheek disease
D. Cannot be given to a child with Crohn's disease
E. Should not be given to a child with a history of severe reaction to neomycin

A 1.   **A.** false   **B.** false   **C.** true   **D.** false   **E.** false

Typical febrile convulsions are seen between 6 months and 5 years of age, in 2–5% of children and are generalized tonic or tonic-clonic seizures. There is a family history in up to a third of childern. Drug treatment may not be necessary if the seizure is brief.

A 2.   **A.** true   **B.** true   **C.** false   **D.** false   **E.** false

A low Apgar score at 5 minutes correlates poorly with the development of cerebral palsy, however a low Apgar score at 20 minutes has an observed cerebral palsy rate of nearly 60%. Both seizures and mental retardation are most commonly seen in association with spastic cerebral palsy.

A 3.   **A.** true   **B.** true   **C.** true   **D.** false   **E.** true

Headaches are more common in girls.

A 4.   **A.** false   **B.** false   **C.** true   **D.** true   **E.** false

Absence seizures are not usually associated with developmental delay and have a good prognosis, mostly resolving in adolescence. Typical absence seizures last less than 30 seconds.

A 5.   **A.** true   **B.** false   **C.** true   **D.** false   **E.** false

Waving 'bye-bye' and releasing objects are attained by 1 year of age. A normal infant sits with a bent back at 6 months, and sits well by 7 months.

A 6.   **A.** true   **B.** true   **C.** true   **D.** false   **E.** false

Most children can feed with a spoon by 18 months and do circular scribbles by 2 years.

A 7. **A.** true **B.** true **C.** false **D.** false **E.** false

Jumping is mastered by 3 years, standing on one leg by 4 years and riding a bicycle by 5 years.

A 8. **A.** false **B.** false **C.** false **D.** true **E.** false

A normally developing child would be expected to hop on one leg by 4 years, build a bridge with 3 cubes by 3 years, have 2-word sentences by 2 years, and name colours by 3 years.

A 9. **A.** true **B.** true **C.** true **D.** true **E.** false

The stepping reflex disappears at 2 months.

A 10. **A.** true **B.** true **C.** true **D.** false **E.** true

A child with an IQ of 20–50 has severe learning disability.

A 11. **A.** false **B.** true **C.** false **D.** true **E.** false

Chorionic villous sampling, amniocentesis and percutaneous umbilical blood sampling are all prenatal diagnostic tests.

A 12. **A.** true **B.** true **C.** true **D.** true **E.** true

A 13. **A.** false **B.** true **C.** false **D.** false **E.** true

Down's syndrome infants are hypotonic at birth. Overlapping of the fifth finger over the fourth is a feature of Edwards syndrome.

A 14. **A.** false **B.** true **C.** false **D.** false **E.** true

Turner syndrome infants have the karyotype 45,XO.

A 15. **A.** true **B.** true **C.** true **D.** true **E.** true

A 16. **A.** true **B.** true **C.** true **D.** false **E.** false

Impaired visual acuity is also a feature of orbital cellulitis.

A 17. **A.** true **B.** true **C.** true **D.** false **E.** true

Astigmatism is a difference in the refractive powers of the components of the eye, usually due to irregular curvature of the cornea.

A. false   **B.** true   **C.** false   **D.** false   **E.** true

After splenectomy there is a thrombocytosis. Prophylactic penicillin should be continued for life. Prior to splenectomy children should have triple vaccination to pneumococcus, *Haemophilus influenzae* and meningococcus.

A **19.** **A.** false   **B.** true   **C.** false   **D.** true   **E.** false

Iron deficiency anaemia is common in infants, as they have high requirements for growth and low stores. Formula-fed infants are more at risk because iron is more poorly absorbed than breast milk iron. The most common cause in children is inadequate iron intake.

A **20.** **A.** false   **B.** true   **C.** false   **D.** false   **E.** false

A **21.** **A.** false   **B.** false   **C.** false   **D.** false   **E.** true

Port-wine stains are present at birth and are macular (though with age they can develop papules and nodules). They are only seen in <1% of infants. They do not obscure vision directly, but if they involve the eyelid, they may be associated with congenital glaucoma and should be seen by an ophthalmologist.

A **22.** **A.** false   **B.** true   **C.** false   **D.** false   **E.** false

Scabies infection is due to infestation with the mite *Sarcoptes scabiei*. The rash is of itchy papules and vesicles, and sometimes burrows are visible. In infants, the wrists, feet (particularly the lateral border), head, face and neck are typically affected. In older children, the finger and toe webs, wrists and genitalia are affected in particular. All close contacts should be treated. An itchy rash may persist for 2–3 weeks after adequate treatment.

A **23.** **A.** true   **B.** true   **C.** true   **D.** true   **E.** true

Almost any lumbosacral cutaneous abnormality lying in the midline may indicate occult spinal dysraphism including abnormalities of pigmentation, vascular anomalies, pits and sinuses, skin tags, lipoma, hypertrichosis and aplasia cutis congenita.

A 24. A. false **B.** false **C.** true **D.** true **E.** true

Phenylketonuria is an amino acid metabolism disorder, resulting from a deficiency or absence of the enzyme phenylalanine hydroxylase which metabolizes phenylalanine.

A 25. A. true **B.** false **C.** false **D.** true **E.** true

Substitution with a cow's milk hydrolysate milk is the treatment of choice (e.g. Pregestimil, Nutramigen, Pepti-Junoir, or an elemental milk such as Neocate). UTIs are a recognized cause of GOR and should be looked for. A reflux index less than 10% in infancy and less than 6% thereafter is still considered 'normal', although it must be stressed that the trace and event markers must be looked at and correlated.

A 26. A. true **B.** true **C.** true **D.** true **E.** true

A Kasai porto-enterostomy should take place before 60 days of age to prevent chronic cholestatic liver disease ensuing.

A 27. A. true **B.** true **C.** true **D.** false **E.** false

Breast-fed infants have fewer episodes of otitis media, and respiratory and gastrointestinal infections than formula-fed infants. Immunological protection, particularly secretory IgA is transferred in breast milk.

A 28. A. true **B.** false **C.** true **D.** false **E.** false

Innocent murmurs are soft and do not radiate. A venous hum is continous (therefore having a diastolic component).

A 29. A. true **B.** true **C.** true **D.** false **E.** false

Feeding is poor and associated with sweating. Peripheral oedema is not a feature.

A 30. A. false **B.** false **C.** true **D.** false **E.** false

A 31. A. true **B.** false **C.** true **D.** false **E.** false

Urinary tract infection occurs in approximately 1% of boys and 3% of girls. It may present with asymptomatic bacteruria. It is most commonly due to *Escherichia coli* infection.

A **32.** **A.** false   **B.** false   **C.** true   **D.** true   **E.** true

Nocturnal enuresis is seen in 5% of normal 5-year-olds. It is psychological in over 90% of cases. Anticholinergics such as oxybutinin can be used for treatment.

A **33.** **A.** false   **B.** false   **C.** true   **D.** true   **E.** false

Perthes disease is an idiopathic avascular necrosis affecting the femoral head. It most commonly presents in boys aged 4–10 years. A fragmented flattened femoral head often of increased density is seen on plain X-ray.

A **34.** **A.** false   **B.** true   **C.** true   **D.** true   **E.** false

Systemic onset juvenile idiopathic arthritis is a diagnosis of exclusion and defined by arthritis and a recurrent fever, with either a rash, lymphadenopathy, hepatosplenomegaly or serositis. Malignancy is among the differential diagnoses. There is no sex difference.

A **35.** **A.** true   **B.** false   **C.** false   **D.** false   **E.** false

Kawasaki disease is classically characterized by an irritable child, and causes coronary artery aneurysms in up to one-fifth of untreated children. Thrombocytosis is seen during the second and third weeks of illness in particular. All children should be screened with echocardiography, and all are treated with intravenous immunoglobulin in an effort to prevent aneurysms from developing.

A **36.** **A.** false   **B.** true   **C.** false   **D.** false   **E.** true

Congenital dislocation of the hip is associated with oligohydramnios, breech position (particularly extended breech), muscular or neurological problems including spina bifida, and a positive family history. The incidence is 2 in 1000 infants, and it is more common in girls.

A **37.** **A.** true   **B.** false   **C.** false   **D.** false   **E.** true

Osteomyelitis, slipped upper femoral epiphysis and irritable hip all cause a painful limp.

A 38. **A.** false   **B.** true   **C.** false   **D.** false   **E.** false

Otoacoustic emissions are used for neonatal screening. Distraction tests are used from 9 to 24 months. Performance testing (involving conditioning, such as putting balls into a bucket when sounds are heard) is used from 2 to 3 years. Pure tone audiometry can be used from age 3 years.

A 39. **A.** false   **B.** true   **C.** true   **D.** false   **E.** false

A 40. **A.** true   **B.** false   **C.** false   **D.** false   **E.** false

In childhood, asthma is more common in boys. Around half of asthmatic children present by age 3 years, and most present by age 7 years. In only around one-third to a half of children their asthma resolves by adulthood. Almost all children with asthma develop exercise-induced wheeze. A mild asthma attack causes hypocapnoea as the carbon dioxide is blown off secondary to hyperventilation. In a severe attack, the child is unable to blow off the carbon dioxide and hypercapnoea results.

A 41. **A.** true   **B.** false   **C.** true   **D.** true   **E.** false

Late language development and early number development are seen in autism. Developmental stasis or delay is seen in 25–30% of cases. Other features include repetitive play, lone play, limited eye contact, a fascination with movement and detail, but a poor concentration span. The diagnosis is usually made between 2–3 years, but features are recognizable from at least 1 year.

A 42. **A.** true   **B.** true   **C.** true   **D.** true   **E.** true

Bulimia is very common among adolescent girls. The features are similar to anorexia nervosa, but the weight is usually normal or the child is mildly overweight. Both electrolyte and cardiac abnormalities as in anorexia nervosa may be seen.

A 43. **A.** false   **B.** false   **C.** false   **D.** true   **E.** false

Night terrors (as opposed to nightmares) occur during deep non-REM stage IV sleep. The child sits up and screams and may stare and sweat profusely. They last from only a few seconds to minutes at most and are not easily recalled. If the child is awoken, they can be difficult to settle back to sleep, otherwise they tend to go back to sleep rapidly.

A 44. **A.** false **B.** true **C.** true **D.** true **E.** true

Amniocentesis is used for the antenatal detection of major trisomies and sex chromosome aneuploidies. Other rarer mutations can also be screened for. In addition, enzyme analysis for certain inborn errors of metabolism and tests for congenital infection using PCR to search for viral particle DNA can be done.

A 45. **A.** false **B.** false **C.** false **D.** true **E.** false

Trisomy 21 and Trisomy 18 both cause a decrease in maternal serum alpha-fetoprotein levels. Multiple pregnancy, open spina bifida, fetomaternal haemorrhage and polycystic kidney disease all cause an increase in maternal serum alpha-fetoprotein levels.

A 46. **A.** false **B.** true **C.** true **D.** true **E.** true

Brown fat metabolism and muscular activity are the main mechanisms used by neonates to maintain heat. Sweating is present, though less than in adults.

A 47. **A.** false **B.** true **C.** true **D.** true **E.** false

Sudden infant death syndrome is most common at 2–4 months of age, and is unlikely to occur over the age of 6 months. The risk is reduced by putting the infant to sleep supine, avoiding overheating, using blankets with holes in them and avoiding smoking during pregnancy and while in the house.

A 48. **A.** true **B.** false **C.** true **D.** false **E.** false

The red reflex should be present: if it is white, then there is cause for concern. Cyanosis of the tongue indicates central cyanosis. A bulging anterior fontanelle indicates raised intracranial pressure. Peeling of the hands and feet is common and often indicates post-maturity.

A 49. **A.** false **B.** false **C.** false **D.** true **E.** false

Vitamin K is necessary for the clotting factors II, VII, IX and X. It is recommended for all neonates to prevent haemorrhagic disease of the newborn. Breast-fed infants are more at risk than bottle-fed infants.

A 50. **A.** false **B.** true **C.** true **D.** false **E.** false

Children with type 2 diabetes mellitus are usually overweight, and have a positive family history of the disease. Acanthosis nigricans (pigmented velvety skin changes in the axillae) is also usually present. Presentation is usually with glycosuria without ketonuria, and with mild or no polyuria and polydipsia, and usually no weight loss. Islet cell antibodies are generally absent unlike in type 1 diabetes mellitus.

A 51. **A.** true **B.** true **C.** true **D.** true **E.** true

Hyperthyroidism may cause either delayed or precocious puberty, the mechanism of which is not well understood. Cardiac features include tachycardia, hypertension, palpitations, dyspnoea, atrial fibrillation and cardiomegaly.

A 52. **A.** false **B.** false **C.** false **D.** true **E.** false

In short stature due to constitutional delay, height and weight are usually on the same low percentile, but head circumference is on a higher percentile. The bone age tends to be delayed by 2–4 years and advances in parallel with the chronological age. There is usually a parental or sibling history of similar constitutional delay.

A 53. **A.** false **B.** true **C.** true **D.** false **E.** false

Gynaecomastia occurs in up to two-thirds of boys to some degree. It usually resolves within 6 months to 3 years. No treatment other than reassurance is necessary in the majority of cases.
Physiological pubertal gynaecomastia may involve one breast, or both but at different rates of growth.

A 54. **A.** true **B.** true **C.** false **D.** false **E.** false

Chloramphenicol causes the 'grey baby syndrome', particularly in neonates with immature liver metabolism (abdominal distension, pallid cyanosis and circulatory collapse). The red man syndrome is caused by vancomycin.

A. false **B.** true **C.** false **D.** true **E.** false

Sodium valproate is given for juvenile myoclonic epilepsy. Carbamazepine is an enzyme inducer. It can cause reversible alopecia.

A 56. **A.** false **B.** false **C.** true **D.** true **E.** false

Kawasaki disease is an arteritis of unknown cause. The clinical features are the presence of a fever of >38.5 °C for more than 5 days, and four of the following: conjunctivitis (bilateral, non-suppurative), lymphadenopathy (cervical, greater than 1.5 cm size), polymorphous rash, lips or oral mucosa changes (cracked red lips or erythema of the oropharynx) and changes of the extremities (erythema and oedema of palms and soles, then peeling from fingertips). Fewer than four features are needed for diagnosis if coronary artery aneurysms are detected. In addition 'incomplete' cases may evolve into 'complete' cases. In 20–40% of cases coronary artery aneurysms develop. Treatment is with both intravenous immunoglobulin and aspirin.

A 57. **A.** false **B.** false **C.** false **D.** true **E.** true

Mumps infection is most common in the winter and spring. Most commonly, the parotid glands are affected and occasionally also the submandibular glands, but rarely the latter alone. Mumps is a common cause of viral meningitis, and encephalitis occurs in approximately 1 in 5000 cases.

A 58. **A.** false **B.** false **C.** false **D.** false **E.** true

Measles has a 1- to 2-week incubation period, and begins with a prodrome of high fever, conjunctivitis and coryzal symptoms. Koplik's spots appear on the buccal mucosa before the rash, which begins behind the ears and on the face, spreading to the body.

A 59. **A.** false **B.** false **C.** false **D.** false **E.** true

Chicken pox is a DNA herpes virus. The incubation period is 2–3 weeks. Young children often have no prodromal illness, unlike older children who have a mild prodrome with fever for 2–3 days. Pneumonia is a common complication in adults but not children. Congenital infection can cause congenital bands, atrophic limbs, skin defects and mental retardation. If maternal infection is acquired close to delivery, the infant may be born with chicken pox lesions.

A **60.** **A.** false **B.** true **C.** false **D.** false **E.** true

Hand, foot and mouth disease is due to Coxsackie A or B or enterovirus infection. It can be transmitted via the faecal-oral route or by direct contact. It is most commonly seen in pre-school children. The rash consists of vesicles on the palms, soles and in the mouth and papules (but not vesicles) are commonly seen on the buttocks.

A **61.** **A.** false **B.** false **C.** true **D.** false **E.** false

Whooping cough is due to *Bordetella pertussis* infection, is spread by droplet infection, and has a 7- to 14-day incubation period. Antibiotic therapy (erythromycin) of the child and close contacts prevents spread but does not alter the course of the infection. The paroxysms of coughing can result in conjunctival petechiae, epistaxis and other symptoms including rectal prolapse, inguinal hernia and phrenulum tear.

A **62.** **A.** false **B.** false **C.** true **D.** false **E.** false

An acute febrile illness is a temporary contraindication to childhood vaccination. A mild illness without systemic upset such as a cold is not a contraindication. Severe local reaction to the previous dose is no longer a contraindication to further doses.

A **63.** **A.** true **B.** false **C.** false **D.** true **E.** true

If the tuberculin test is positive this indicates either the child has TB (and should be treated for TB) or is immune (dependent on clinical history). The BCG is a live virus, and therefore should not be given to children with malignant conditions. Neither should it be given if there is a widespread infective skin condition, or to an HIV positive child.

A **64.** **A.** false **B.** true **C.** false **D.** true **E.** false

A child with HIV should be given all vaccines except the BCG and yellow fever. The intramuscular polio vaccine is preferable to the oral polio vaccine as it is inactivated.

A. false **B.** true **C.** true **D.** false **E.** false

Diphtheria vaccine is a toxoid. It should not be given to a child with an acute febrile illness (such as slapped cheek disease) or to a child who has had an anaphylactic reaction to a previous dose.

Exam 1

Answers

Q 1. Migraine in childhood

   A. Most frequently presents with an aura
   B. May occur with an aura but no headache
   C. Is often associated with paraesthesia
   D. May be triggered by certain foods
   E. Is not relieved by simple analgesia

Q 2. The parents of a child who has had a typical febrile convulsion should be advised

   A. To keep the temperature low during febrile illnesses
   B. Rectal diazepam should be given if the fit lasts longer than 15 minutes
   C. There are usually no further episodes during the same febrile illness
   D. Prophylactic anti-epileptic drugs should be commenced
   E. The risk of epilepsy is the same as for the general population

Q 3. Cerebral palsy

   A. Is a disorder of movement and posture due to a progressive lesion in the developing brain
   B. Is associated with hearing loss in about a third of cases
   C. Affects approximately 2 in 1000 live births in the UK
   D. Is usually associated with learning impairment
   E. Is rarely associated with epilepsy

Q 4. Absence seizures

   A. Have a short post-ictal phase
   B. Require no treatment
   C. May involve eyelid fluttering
   D. Are seen in 10% of children
   E. Have a typical 1 per second spike and wave EEG

Q 5. A normal newborn

A. Has marked head lag when pulled up to sit
B. Can follow a face
C. Will startle to noise
D. Can smile responsively
E. Has hand regard

Q 6. A normal 3-month-old infant

A. Has a pincer grasp
B. Reaches for objects
C. Pushes up with their arms when prone
D. Babbles
E. Has good head control

Q 7. A normal 18-month-old child would be expected to

A. Pull to stand
B. Build a 6-cube tower
C. Draw circular scribbles
D. Have 2-word sentences
E. Feed themselves with a spoon

Q 8. The following are concerning signs of developmental delay

A. Not sitting unsupported by 6 months
B. Unable to walk by 14 months
C. Not smiling responsively by 8 weeks
D. No good eye contact by 3 months
E. No single words by 1 year

Q 9. The following are correct

A. The forward parachute appears at 2 months
B. The Landau reflex appears at 2 months
C. The asymmetric tonic neck reflex is present from birth
D. The Moro reflex appears at 1 month
E. The palmar grasp disappears at 3–4 months

Q 10. The following are signs of possible developmental delay

A. Moro reflex present at 6 months
B. Not crawling by 1 year
C. Not sitting unsupported by 1 year

D. Not smiling responsively by 2 months

E. Hand preference by 1 year

Q 11. Regarding Down's syndrome

A. Most cases are the result of non-disjunction

B. Most Down's syndrome infants are born to women aged over 40 years

C. An average 30-year-old woman has a risk of 1 in 1000 of conceiving a Down's syndrome child

D. The risk of recurrence is 10% if neither parent has a translocation

E. Girls are more commonly affected than boys

Q 12. The following are features of Turner syndrome

A. Visuo-spacial difficulties

B. A short webbed neck

C. Growth hormone responsive short stature

D. Seizures

E. A wide fontanelle

Q 13. In autosomal recessive disorders

A. Cases are seen in successive generations

B. The offspring of two carrier parents have a 50% chance of inheriting the condition

C. The conditions are often structural defects

D. Consanguinity increases the chances of the disorder being expressed

E. A single allele exerts an effect

Q 14. In Klinefelter's syndrome

A. The karyotype is 47,XYY

B. An estimated 1 in 2000 males are affected

C. Behavioural difficulties may present

D. Secondary infertility is a feature

E. The phenotype is tall and slim

Q 15. The following are true

A. Neonates have 6/6 acuity

B. Binocular vision is present from birth

C. Depth perception begins at 4–6 weeks

D. Any untreated interference with focusing on objects during the first 7 years of life can cause amblyopia

E. A squint in a neonate can be normal

Q 16. The following tests of visual acuity are correctly age-matched

A. Picks up hundreds and thousands – 8 months

B. Face fixation – birth

C. Picks up a raisin – 6 months

D. Identifies pictures of reducing size – 1 year

E. Fixes and follows a face through 180 degrees, 90 cm away – 6 weeks

Q 17. Colour blindness

A. Can affect girls

B. Usually involves difficulty distinguishing the colours red, green and blue

C. Is transmitted as an X-linked recessive trait

D. Of new onset could indicate optic nerve damage

E. Is often associated with photophobia

Q 18. The following are true regarding iron

A. Dried fruit and nuts are rich in iron

B. Vitamin C enhances iron absorption

C. High fibre foods increase iron absorption

D. Iron from cow's milk is easily absorbed

E. Baby cereals are iron enriched

Q 19. Sickle cell anaemia

A. Is associated with failure to thrive

B. Can cause renal failure

C. Is seen in Mediterraneans

D. Is associated with splenomegaly in infancy

E. Is managed with recommended daily folic acid

Q 20. Neurofibromatosis type 1 is the most likely diagnosis in a 4-year-old girl with

A. 2 Lisch nodules of the iris

B. More than five café-au-lait macules above 5 mm in size and axillary freckles

C. More than four café-au-lait macules above 5 mm in size

D. A first-degree relative with neurofibromatosis type 1

E. Three neurofibromas

Q 21. Haemangiomas

A. Usually appear after 2–3 months

B. Are seen in around 1% of infants

C. Worsen with time becoming larger and darker over the years

D. Are usually treated with a pulsed dye laser

E. Are most common on the head and neck

Q 22. Tinea capitis

A. Requires hair pluckings to be taken for diagnostic confirmation

B. Can be treated with topical antifungal treatment

C. Presents as a smooth annular area of alopecia

D. Is most prevalent in Asian children in the UK

E. Is most commonly due to *Trichophyton mentagrophytes*

Q 23. Pityriasis versicolor

A. Is inherited in autosomal dominant fashion

B. Is most common in infants

C. Is only present in the summer

D. Is due to a yeast infection

E. Is associated with inflammatory bowel disease

Q 24. Galactosaemia

A. Presents around the age of 1 year

B. Is a cause of developmental delay

C. Can be diagnosed by a positive urine clinistix

D. Is managed by a phenylalanine-free diet for life

E. Causes hepatosplenomegaly

Q 25. The following are true of jaundice occurring in the first month of life in term infants

A. Physiological jaundice occurs in only 20% of infants

B. Physiological jaundice usually lasts until the fourth week of life

C. Jaundice occurring with hypothyroidism can be conjugated or unconjugated

D. Breast-feeding should be discontinued if this is determined to be the cause after 14 days of age

E. Breast milk jaundice lasts for the first 4 months of life

Q 26. **Recognized complications of Crohn's disease include**

A. Toxic megacolon

B. Vitamin B12 deficiency

C. Renal calculi

D. Caseating granulomas

E. Eventual diminished adult height if testicular volume is 5–10 ml at 17 years of age

Q 27. **The following maternal drugs or conditions are relative or absolute contraindications to breast-feeding**

A. Metronidazole

B. Phenylketonuria

C. Maternal tuberculosis

D. Maternal cocaine abuse

E. Lithium

Q 28. **The following conditions and congenital heart defects are associated**

A. Turner syndrome – ventricular septal defect

B. Down's syndrome – ventricular septal defect

C. Noonan syndrome – tetralogy of Fallot

D. Turner syndrome – coarctation of the aorta

E. Marfan syndrome – aortic regurgitation

Q 29. **With a ventricular septal defect**

A. The murmur may be asymptomatic

B. Endocarditis is not a risk

C. It is the most common form of structural congenital heart disease

D. The murmur is pansystolic

E. Surgical repair is always necessary

Q 30. **To parents of an infant born with structural congenital heart disease (CHD), the best advice regarding the recurrence risk for future children is**

A. There is no increased risk for future children

B. There is a 3% risk of a future child having CHD

C. There is a 10% risk of a future child having CHD
D. There is a 25% risk of a future child having CHD
E. Antenatal diagnosis is not possible

Q 31. Regarding urinary continence

A. Daytime continence is achieved in half of children by the age of 2.5 years
B. Night-time continence is achieved in 95% of children by age 5 years
C. 2–3% of 10-year-olds have nocturnal enuresis
D. Girls achieve continence sooner than boys on average
E. Urinalysis is essential in the investigation of nocturnal enuresis

Q 32. The following advice should be given to parents of a child to prevent further urinary tract infections

A. Avoid constipation
B. Girls should wipe themselves from back to front after micturition
C. Keep fluid intake low
D. Prophylactic antibiotics are necessary until puberty
E. No renal investigation is necessary after one urinary tract infection

Q 33. Septic arthritis

A. Is most common among school age children
B. Usually results from haematogenous spread
C. May be multifocal in neonates
D. Causes a pseudoparesis of the involved joint
E. May be caused by enterococci

Q 34. Reactive arthritis

A. Predominantly affects the elbow joint
B. Is a feature of rheumatic fever
C. May be secondary to *Shigella* infection
D. Is managed conservatively
E. May become recurrent

Q 35. Scheuermann's disease

A. Is an osteochondritis affecting the pelvis
B. May be painless

C. Causes a wedging of the vertebrae

D. Is idiopathic

E. Is usually managed with surgical intervention

Q 36. Irritable hip

A. Is self-limiting

B. Has a normal range of hip movement on examination

C. Is an uncommon cause of acute hip pain in children

D. Is associated with gastrointestinal illness

E. Is managed with rest and anti-inflammatory drugs

Q 37. A pulled elbow

A. Is always tender

B. Is seen in school age children

C. Is not visible on X-ray

D. May present with a pseudoparalysis of the affected forearm

E. Is uncommon

Q 38. Regarding hearing the following would be cause for concern in newborns

A. A family history of deafness

B. Birth weight below 1.5 kg

C. Congenital toxoplasmosis

D. Neonatal jaundice requiring phototherapy

E. Turner syndrome

Q 39. In a child with suspected foreign body inhalation the most useful investigation would be

A. A plain chest X-ray

B. An inspiratory and expiratory chest X-ray

C. A chest CT

D. A chest MRI

E. Rigid bronchoscopy

Q 40. The following are symptoms of obstructive sleep apnoea syndrome

A. Night sweats

B. Nocturnal cough

C. Enuresis

D. Altered personality
E. Evening headaches

Q 41. The following are features of anorexia nervosa

A. Constipation
B. Fast relaxing reflexes
C. Hypothermia
D. Short QT interval
E. Terminal hairs on face and body

Q 42. Depression is associated with

A. Apathy
B. Attention deficit hyperactivity disorder
C. Faltering growth
D. An increase in prevalence in girls pre-adolescence
E. Conduct disorder

Q 43. The following are features of functional abdominal pain

A. Poor school performance
B. Equal sex ratio
C. Most common in adolescence
D. Para-umbilical pain
E. Change in bowel habit

Q 44. Infants of diabetic mothers are at increased risk of

A. Organomegaly
B. Hydrops fetalis
C. Renal vein thrombosis
D. Congenital heart disease
E. Caudal regression syndrome

Q 45. The following fetal conditions may be diagnosed by the 20-week anomaly scan

A. Gastroschisis
B. Diaphragmatic hernia
C. Hydrops fetalis
D. Cleft lip
E. Hydronephrosis

Q 46. Erb's palsy

    A. Is a common injury to the lower roots of the brachial plexus

    B. Causes a wrist drop

    C. May be associated with a Horner's syndrome

    D. Usually spontaneously improves over a few months

    E. Affects 1 in 200 newborns

Q 47. In normal newborns

    A. They usually turn their heads to the left

    B. The umbilical cord may remain attached for 1 month

    C. The umbilical cord usually coils clockwise

    D. Cephalhaematoma is present in up to 2.5% of births

    E. They may have ankle clonus

Q 48. Regarding apparent life-threatening events in infants

    A. There are often no other significant features in addition to the event

    B. They may be caused by gastro-oesophageal reflux

    C. They may be due to viral infection

    D. A cause must be found for diagnosis

    E. There is no benefit to teaching the parents resuscitation skills

Q 49. Microcephaly in the newborn may be caused by

    A. Hypothyroidism

    B. Craniosynostosis

    C. Maternal smoking in pregnancy

    D. Raised intracranial pressure

    E. Maternal alcohol abuse

Q 50. Diabetes insipidus

    A. Is due to insufficiency of somatomedin

    B. May present with faltering growth

    C. Causes palmar hyperpigmentation

    D. Is unlikely if morning urine is dilute

    E. Is a cause of glycosuria

Q 51. Glycosylated haemoglobin (HbA1c)

    A. Is the fraction of haemoglobin to which glucose has been non-enzymatically attached in the circulation

B. Represents the average blood glucose concentration over the previous 4 weeks
C. Level is zero in normal children
D. Continues to form reversibly during the red blood cells' lifespan
E. Levels may spuriously be elevated in thalassaemia

Q 52. The following conditions may cause precocious puberty

A. Hypothyroidism
B. Klinefelter's syndrome
C. Hydrocephalus
D. Neurofibromatosis
E. Ovarian tumour

Q 53. Regarding growth patterns

A. The rate of linear growth decreases in infancy after the age of 1 year
B. The pubertal growth spurt begins at age 11 years in girls on average
C. The pubertal growth spurt begins at age 12 years in boys on average
D. The peak growth rate in boys occurs at age 12 years
E. Girls generally stop growing later than boys

Q 54. Phenytoin

A. Causes hypertrichosis
B. Displays zero-order kinetics
C. Causes dose-dependent vertigo
D. Results in intellectual deterioration
E. Is a potassium channel blocker

Q 55. The following antibiotics should be avoided or used with extreme caution in hepatic failure

A. Erythromycin
B. Tetracycline
C. Rifampicin
D. Chloramphenicol
E. Clindamycin

Q 56. **Complications of measles**

    A. Are more common in children with vitamin A deficiency
    B. Include an abnormal EEG in up to 50% of cases
    C. Include otitis media
    D. Include sterility in males
    E. Include hepatitis

Q 57. **Treatment with varicella zoster immunoglobulin (VZIG) for children exposed to chicken pox is indicated for**

    A. Children on immunosuppressive drugs
    B. Children with congenital immunodeficiency
    C. Neonates of mothers with maternal infection 2 weeks prior to delivery
    D. Neonates of mothers with maternal infection 1 week post-delivery
    E. Children on high dose steroids in the previous 3 months

Q 58. **Mumps infection**

    A. Has an incubation period of 5–7 days
    B. Usually causes painless parotid gland swelling
    C. Is infectious from 6 days before the onset of parotid gland swelling
    D. Is spread by droplet route
    E. Can cause hepatitis

Q 59. **Whooping cough**

    A. Is caused by the Gram-negative bacillus *Bartonella pertussis*
    B. Has an incubation period of 2–3 weeks
    C. Can be rapidly curtailed with prompt erythromycin treatment
    D. Is highly infectious during the paroxysmal stage
    E. Can cause rectal prolapse

Q 60. **Rubella**

    A. Has a 7-day incubation period
    B. Has a prodrome of rhinitis and fever
    C. Is a cause of palatal petechiae
    D. Usually causes symptomatic disease in children over 5 years of age
    E. Can cause a thrombocythaemia

Q 61. Threadworms

A. Cause pruritis ani, mostly in the mornings
B. Are always symptomatic in children
C. Can cause anaemia
D. Are a cause of faltering growth
E. Should be treated with albendazole

Q 62. The following are contraindications to childhood vaccination

A. Previous history of pertussis
B. Mother is in the first trimester of pregnancy
C. Systemic upset with high fever to previous dose
D. Anaphylaxis to previous dose
E. Recent tonsillectomy

Q 63. The MMR vaccine can be given to a child with

A. Severe allergy to neomycin
B. Autism
C. Wilms' tumour
D. Congenital immunodeficiency
E. The snuffles

Q 64. Recommended minimal interval times between vaccines are

A. 4 weeks between any live vaccines not given simultaneously
B. 6 weeks between first and second Hib
C. 6 weeks between the BCG and the first DTP, polio, Hib and meningococcal C
D. 1 year between the DTP and first MMR
E. 1 month between DTP and meningococcal C conjugate

Q 65. Roseola infantum

A. Is caused by an echovirus
B. Is usually asymptomatic
C. Is the cause of approximately one-third of febrile convulsions in children under 2 years old
D. Is characterized by bright red cheeks and a truncal macular erythema
E. Causes severe anaemia in congenital infection

A 1.   **A.** false **B.** true **C.** false **D.** true **E.** false

Migraine usually presents without an aura, and is only occasionally associated with paraesthesia. Foods that can trigger migraine include chocolate, cheese and food colourings. Alcohol is also a trigger. Simple analgesia may be sufficient, however anti-emetics and other medication (e.g. 5-HT agonists in those over 12 years old, or beta-blockers – except in asthmatics) may be needed.

A 2.   **A.** true **B.** false **C.** true **D.** false **E.** false

Rectal diazepam should be given for seizures greater than 5 minutes. Further fits occur in the same febrile illness in around 15% of cases only. Most children have a simple febrile convulsion and further treatment with anti-epileptic medication is not necessary. The risk of epilepsy in children who have had a febrile convulsion is 1%, and the population risk is 0.5%.

A 3.   **A.** false **B.** false **C.** true **D.** true **E.** false

Cerebral palsy is a disorder of movement and posture due to a *non-progressive* lesion in the developing brain. There is associated deafness in about one-fifth of cases, and epilepsy in over one-third of cases.

A 4.   **A.** false **B.** false **C.** true **D.** false **E.** false

Absence seizures have no post-ictal phase. They may require anti-epileptic medication. The EEG shows a 3 per second spike and wave pattern.

A 5.   **A.** true **B.** true **C.** true **D.** false **E.** false

A 6-week-old infant will smile responsively. A 3-month-old infant has hand regard.

A 6. **A.** false   **B.** true   **C.** true   **D.** true   **E.** true

Pincer grasp develops at 9–14 months.

A 7. **A.** true   **B.** false   **C.** false   **D.** false   **E.** true

A normal 18-month-old child can build a 3-cube tower. Circular scribbles and 2-word sentences develop by 2 years of age.

A 8. **A.** false   **B.** false   **C.** true   **D.** true   **E.** false

Infants may be able to sit unsupported from 6 months and by 9 months at the latest. Walking is very variable, and particularly if bottom-shuffling, may be up to 18 months. Single words said with meaning usually develop from 1 year and by 18 months at the latest.

A 9. **A.** false   **B.** false   **C.** true   **D.** false   **E.** true

The forward parachute appears at 5–6 months, the Landau reflex from 3–6 months. The Moro reflex is present from birth.

A 10. **A.** true   **B.** true   **C.** true   **D.** true   **E.** true

A 11. **A.** true   **B.** false   **C.** true   **D.** false   **E.** false

The individual risk of having a Down's syndrome infant is higher for women over 40 years, however most Down's syndrome infants are born to younger women as there are more infants born to this age group. If neither parent has a translocation, the risk of a second Down's child is estimated at 1%. Girls and boys are equally affected.

A 12. **A.** true   **B.** true   **C.** true   **D.** false   **E.** false

A 13. **A.** false   **B.** false   **C.** false   **D.** true   **E.** false

In autosomal recessive disorders the inheritance pattern is horizontal (i.e. it is seen in multiple siblings but not the parents). The offspring of two carrier parents have a 50% chance of being a carrier and a 25% chance of inheriting the condition. Both alleles need to carry the mutation for the disease to be expressed.

A 14. **A.** false   **B.** false   **C.** true   **D.** false   **E.** true

Klinefelter's syndrome karyotype is 47,XXY. Approximately 1 in 500 males are affected. Primary infertility is present.

A. false   **B.** false   **C.** false   **D.** true   **E.** true

Neonates have approximately 6/200 vision. Binocular vision develops during the first 3–6 months of age, and depth perception from 6–8 months.

A 16. **A.** false   **B.** true   **C.** false   **D.** false   **E.** false

A child will pick up hundreds and thousands by 1 year, raisins by 10 months, and will identify pictures of reducing size at 2 years. At 6 weeks, an infant fixes and follows a face through 90 degrees, but not to the midline until 3 months of age.

A 17. **A.** true   **B.** true   **C.** false   **D.** true   **E.** false

The different types of colour blindness have different inheritance patterns. Blue colour blindness is transmitted by autosomal dominant inheritance. Both optic nerve and retinal disease can cause a change in colour vision. Total colour vision defect with photophobia, nystagmus and defective visual acuity is a rare occurrence.

A 18. **A.** true   **B.** true   **C.** false   **D.** false   **E.** true

High fibre foods decrease iron absorption. Iron from cow's milk is poorly absorbed.

A 19. **A.** true   **B.** true   **C.** true   **D.** true   **E.** true

A 20. **A.** false   **B.** true   **C.** false   **D.** false   **E.** false

The diagnosis of neurofibromatosis type 1 in a 4-year-old requires at least 2 signs from the following list:

1. Greater than five café-au-lait macules larger than 5 mm in size
2. Axillary freckles
3. At least two neurofibromas or one plexiform neurofibroma
4. At least two Lisch nodules of the iris
5. A specified bone lesion
6. Optic glioma
7. A first-degree relative with neurofibromatosis

Exam 2

Answers

A **21.** **A.** false **B.** false **C.** false **D.** false **E.** true

Haemangiomas usually appear during the first 2–3 weeks of life, and are seen in about 1 in 20 (5%) of infants. They enlarge over a period of months and then begin to slowly involute. They do not require treatment unless they are complicated, which may then involve oral steroids or surgery. A pulsed dye laser is used for ulcerated haemangiomas.

A **22.** **A.** false **B.** false **C.** false **D.** false **E.** false

Tinea capitis presents as annular patches of hair loss with superficial scale. There may be several patches, or a moth-eaten appearance in extensive infection. It is most commonly seen in the UK in Afro-Caribbean children. It is usually due to *Trichophyton tonsurans*. Systemic treatment is necessary for scalp infection.

A **23.** **A.** false **B.** false **C.** false **D.** true **E.** false

Pityriasis versicolor is a common yeast infection caused by *Pityrosporum ovale*. It is most common in adolescents and young adults, and becomes more obvious in the summer when the individual is suntanned and the patches are relatively hypopigmented.

A **24.** **A.** false **B.** true **C.** false **D.** false **E.** true

Galactosaemia presents during infancy after milk feeds are commenced. The urine clinitest (for reducing substances) is positive, but the clinistix (for glucose) is negative. The definitive diagnosis is made by a blood enzyme assay. Management is by a lactose- and galactose-free diet.

A **25.** **A.** false **B.** false **C.** true **D.** false **E.** false

Physiological jaundice occurs in up to 65% of term and 80% of preterm infants, and only usually lasts to days 5–7 of life. Breast milk jaundice is a diagnosis of exclusion and can last for the first 4 weeks of life, is unconjugated, poorly understood and does not require cessation of breast-feeding as it very rarely causes any pathology. Hydration and adequate milk production should be ascertained.

A 26. **A.** false **B.** true **C.** true **D.** false **E.** false

Toxic megacolon is a feature of ulcerative colitis. Terminal ileal involvement may impair vitamin B12 absorption. Non-caseating granulomas occur. Until testicular volume reaches 20 ml there is potential for increased height.

Leichtner A, Jackson W, Grand R. Chapter 27. In *Pediatric Gastrointestinal Disease*. Ed. Walker A *et al.* St Louis: Mosby, 1996.

A 27. **A.** true **B.** true **C.** true **D.** true **E.** true

In addition breast-feeding is contraindicated if there are active herpes lesions on the breast, with maternal narcotic abuse, and if the mother is on bromocriptine (this suppresses lactation).

A 28. **A.** false **B.** true **C.** false **D.** true **E.** true

Down's syndrome is associated with atrial and ventricular septal defects, atrioventricular septal defects and a patent ductus arteriosus.

A 29. **A.** true **B.** false **C.** true **D.** true **E.** false

Prophylaxis against endocarditis must be taken when necessary in a child with a ventricular septal defect. Surgical repair may not be necessary as some defects will close spontaneously during the first few years of life.

A 30. **A.** false **B.** true **C.** false **D.** false **E.** false

A 31. **A.** true **B.** true **C.** true **D.** true **E.** true

Urinalysis to check for an undiagnosed urinary tract infection or diabetes is important in the assessment of nocturnal enuresis.

A 32. **A.** true **B.** false **C.** false **D.** false **E.** false

Girls should wipe themselves from front to back after micturition, and fluid intake should be kept high. Further investigations of renal tract anatomy and function are necessary after a urinary tract infection has been diagnosed in a child. Prophylactic antibiotics are only necessary until those investigations have excluded renal damage, anatomical or functional pathology.

A 33.   **A.** false   **B.** true   **C.** true   **D.** true   **E.** true

Septic arthritis is most common in infants below the age of 2 years. The most common infective agents are *Staphylococcus aureus* and streptococci.

A 34.   **A.** false   **B.** true   **C.** true   **D.** true   **E.** true

Reactive arthritis is a viral and post-infectious arthritis seen in acute rheumatic fever and following both gastrointestinal and genitourinary infections. It predominantly affects the lower limb joints. It may last from weeks to months and recurrences over several years occur.

A 35.   **A.** false   **B.** true   **C.** true   **D.** true   **E.** false

Scheuermann's disease is an idiopathic osteochondritis of the spine causing wedging of the vertebrae and kyphosis. It may be either painful or painless. It is generally self-limiting and conservative treatment is used.

A 36.   **A.** true   **B.** false   **C.** false   **D.** true   **E.** true

Irritable hip is a transient tenosynovitis associated with both bacterial and viral illnesses, and is a diagnosis of exclusion. It is a common cause of acute hip pain in children aged 2–12 years.

A 37.   **A.** false   **B.** true   **C.** false   **D.** true   **E.** false

Pulled elbow is a common injury of toddlers caused by a rapid pull on the child's arm. There is a dislocation of the radial head though the annular ligament which is visible on plain X-ray.

A 38.   **A.** true   **B.** true   **C.** true   **D.** false   **E.** false

Severe neonatal jaundice (levels requiring exchange transfusion) can cause sensorineural deafness in infants.

A 39.   **A.** false   **B.** true   **C.** false   **D.** false   **E.** false

A 40.   **A.** true   **B.** false   **C.** true   **D.** true   **E.** false

Obstructive sleep apnoea causes frequent night-time awakening and hypercapnoea. These result in daytime sleepiness, learning problems, personality changes and morning headaches.

A. true   **B.** false   **C.** true   **D.** false   **E.** false

In anorexia nervosa the reflexes are slow relaxing, there is hypothermia, bradycardia and hypotension with a pronounced postural drop and prolonged QT interval. There are vellus hairs on the face and body.

A **42.** **A.** true   **B.** true   **C.** true   **D.** false   **E.** true

Depression is more common in boys during pre-adolescence but more common in girls during adolescence. It is associated with other behavioural disturbances (e.g. ADHD, conduct disorder, eating disorders), family history of depression, adverse life-events, a dysfunctional family and separation from parents. The features include apathy, faltering growth, protest, despair and detachment in young children. In older children feelings of hopelessness, self-blame, social withdrawal, dropping school performance and recurrent functional pain syndromes are seen.

A **43.** **A.** false   **B.** false   **C.** false   **D.** true   **E.** false

Functional abdominal pain is most common at age 6–9 years, is more common in girls, and is seen in high-achieving personalities who are usually doing well at school, and may be anxious. A change in bowel habit would raise concern of an organic cause.

A **44.** **A.** true   **B.** true   **C.** true   **D.** true   **E.** true

Infants of mothers with diabetes mellitus are usually large for gestational age and have transient neonatal hypoglycaemia. They are also at increased risk of many malformations including caudal regression syndrome, renal vein thrombosis and congenital heart disease.

A **45.** **A.** true   **B.** true   **C.** true   **D.** true   **E.** true

Other conditions diagnosable at the 20-week anomaly scan are hydrocephalus, polycystic kidneys, renal agenesis, congenital heart disease, limb defects and skeletal abnormalities.

A **46.** **A.** false   **B.** false   **C.** true   **D.** true   **E.** false

Erb's palsy is an injury to the upper nerve roots of the brachial plexus, affecting approximately 1 in 2000 infants. It causes the

Exam 2

Answers

'waiter's tip' position of the hand (arm in adduction, elbow extended, internally rotated, forearm pronated and wrist flexed).

A 47. A. false **B.** true **C.** false **D.** true **E.** true

Infants prefer to turn their heads to the right, commencing in utero. The umbilical cord may remain attached in normal infants for around 45 days. The umbilical cord is usually coiled and mostly in an anticlockwise direction. Bilateral ankle clonus can be a normal finding in newborns, particularly if they are hungry or crying.

A 48. A. true **B.** true **C.** true **D.** false **E.** false

Apparent life-threatening events in infants manifest as sudden apnoea, central cyanosis, choking or unresponsiveness often with no other obvious symptoms or signs. It is important to try to find the cause, in particular to exclude serious underlying pathology. There are many causes including sepsis, viral infection, seizures, cardiac events, hypoglycaemia and gastro-oesophageal reflux. However no cause may be found. It is important to teach the parents resuscitation skills in case of a similar future event.

A 49. A. false **B.** true **C.** false **D.** false **E.** true

Congenital hypothyroidism causes large fontanelles with delayed closure. Raised intracranial pressure causes an increased head circumference.

A 50. A. false **B.** true **C.** false **D.** false **E.** false

Diabetes insipidus is caused by insufficiency of vasopressin (antidiuretic hormone, ADH). This results in failure to concentrate urine causing large quantities of dilute urine, polydipsia and dehydration. It can present with failure to thrive due to chronic dehydration, or polydipsia and frequent urination with lots of dilute urine. In an infant, lots of wet nappies may be noticed; difficulty with toilet training in a toddler due to frequent urination or the reappearance of nocturnal enuresis in an older child may also be observed. The diagnosis is unlikely if morning urine is concentrated and serum osmolality is normal. A formal water deprivation test is done to confirm the diagnosis. Glycosuria suggests diabetes mellitus.

A **51.** **A.** true   **B.** false   **C.** false   **D.** false   **E.** true

Glycosylated haemoglobin (HbA1c) is a slow reaction dependent on the blood glucose levels, and continues during the red blood cell's lifespan (approximately 120 days). Because a blood sample contains a mixture of red blood cells of various ages, the HbA1c represents the average blood glucose concentration over the previous 2–3 months. The HbA1c is slightly elevated in normal children.

A **52.** **A.** true   **B.** false   **C.** true   **D.** true   **E.** true

Klinefelter's syndrome is a cause of delayed puberty.

A **53.** **A.** false   **B.** false   **C.** false   **D.** false   **E.** false

In infancy the rate of linear growth begins to decelerate from the age of 2 years. On average the pubertal growth spurt begins at age 9 years for girls and 11 years for boys. The peak rate of growth is at age 13.5 years in boys. Boys generally continue to grow for longer than girls.

A **54.** **A.** false   **B.** true   **C.** true   **D.** true   **E.** false

Phenytoin displays zero-order kinetics. In practical terms this means that above a certain blood level the enzymes involved in its metabolism become saturated, and any further increase in dose results in toxicity with no increase in therapeutic benefit (i.e. a narrow therapeutic window). The mode of action is via inhibiting sodium flux through the Na channels and so blocks repetitive firing of neurons. Side-effects include hirsutism.

A **55.** **A.** true   **B.** true   **C.** true   **D.** true   **E.** true

All of these antibiotics are primarily metabolized or excreted by the liver and should be avoided or used with extreme caution in liver failure.

A **56.** **A.** true   **B.** true   **C.** true   **D.** false   **E.** true

Measles complications are more common in malnourished children, particularly in the presence of vitamin A deficiency. The complications include secondary bacterial pneumonia, bronchitis, hepatitis, myocarditis and encephalomyelitis (rare, although EEG changes are common).

A **57.** **A.** true   **B.** true   **C.** false   **D.** false   **E.** true

Varicella zoster immunoglobulin (VZIG) passive immunization for children exposed to chicken pox is indicated for immunocompromised children (bone marrow transplant patients, congenital immunodeficiency, those on immunosuppressives or high dose steroids within the previous 3 months) and for neonates of mothers infected with varicella from between 5 days pre- and 2 days post-delivery.

A **58.** **A.** false   **B.** false   **C.** true   **D.** true   **E.** true

Mumps has a 2- to 3-week incubation period. The infectious period is from 6 days before the parotid swelling until 9 days after the swelling. There is sometimes a prodrome of fever, headache and earache. The salivary gland swelling is painful. Complications of mumps include meningitis, encephalitis, transient hearing loss, epididymo-orchitis, arthritis and hepatitis.

A **59.** **A.** false   **B.** false   **C.** false   **D.** false   **E.** true

Whooping cough is caused by *Bordetella pertussis*. The incubation period is 1–2 weeks. It is highly infectious during the initial catarrhal stage. Erythromycin treatment reduces infectivity if given early during the illness, however has no effect on the severity of the disease.

A **60.** **A.** false   **B.** false   **C.** true   **D.** true   **E.** false

Rubella has a 14- to 21-day incubation period. The prodrome is of fever, conjunctivitis and cervical lymphadenopathy. It can cause a thrombocytopenia.

A **61.** **A.** false   **B.** false   **C.** false   **D.** false   **E.** false

Threadworms (*Enterobius vermicularum*) cause a pruritis ani particularly at night when the adult worms come out to lay their eggs perianally. They may be asymptomatic. They are treated with mebendazole or piperazine.

A **62.** **A.** false   **B.** false   **C.** false   **D.** true   **E.** false

None of the conditions are contraindications to childhood vaccination, except anaphylaxis to a previous dose.

A. false   **B.** true   **C.** false   **D.** false   **E.** true

The MMR is a live vaccine and therefore cannot be given to immunocompromised children. In addition, severe allergy to neomycin or kanamycin is a contraindication.

A 64.   **A.** false   **B.** false   **C.** false   **D.** false   **E.** false

Live vaccines (which include the BCG) can be given simultaneously or at least 3 weeks apart. The first and second Hib are given at least 4 weeks apart. DTP and meningococcal C conjugate are given as part of the combined infant vaccination at 2, 3 and 4 months.

A 65.   **A.** false   **B.** true   **C.** true   **D.** false   **E.** false

Roseola infantum is caused by herpes virus 6. The clinical features are a high fever and cervical lymphadenopathy with a red macular rash over the face, trunk and arms. Febrile convulsions may occur. Only around one-third of cases are symptomatic, however.

Exam 2

Answers

Q 1. **In a child who presents with recurrent headaches**

A. A full neurological examination including fundoscopy should be done

B. Blood pressure must be checked

C. The mouth should be examined

D. Frontal headaches are a concerning feature

E. Abdominal pain means the headaches are migrainous

Q 2. **Febrile convulsions**

A. Are often due to a viral upper respiratory tract infection

B. Occur after a rapid temperature rise

C. Are more common in girls

D. Are associated with a family history in 50% of cases

E. Should be managed with admission to hospital

Q 3. **Cerebral palsy**

A. Usually presents with abnormal tone in infants

B. Is most commonly caused by birth asphyxia

C. May be due to neonatal jaundice

D. Is divided into four types

E. Is the commonest cause of motor impairment in children

Q 4. **Generalized tonic-clonic seizures**

A. Always have a preceding aura

B. Always have a post-ictal phase

C. Are not always associated with loss of consciousness

D. May have a focal origin

E. Can be treated with sodium valproate

Q 5. **Regarding child development**

A. It is divided into three main areas

B. There is a wide variation in the normal range for walking

C. Hearing problems can result in developmental delay
D. Boys develop bladder control sooner than girls on average
E. The 9-month assessment is usually done by the health visitor

Q 6. **A normal 9-month-old baby will be able to**

A. Transfer objects from one hand to the other
B. Pull to stand
C. Understand no
D. Scribble
E. Build a 3-cube tower

Q 7. **A normal 2-year-old child would be expected to be able to**

A. Draw a circle
B. Jump
C. Kick a ball
D. Undress themselves
E. Use symbolic play

Q 8. **A normal 4-year-old is able to**

A. Draw a triangle
B. Do buttons up
C. Draw a cross
D. Hop
E. Ride a bicycle

Q 9. **The following reflexes/postural responses are present from birth**

A. The lateral propping reflex
B. The stepping reflex
C. The rooting reflex
D. The forward parachute
E. The plantar grasp

Q 10. **The following would be features of concern regarding developmental delay**

A. The pincer grasp not present at 6 months
B. The stepping reflex present at 5 months
C. The Landau reflex not present by 4 months

D. The Moro reflex asymmetrical
E. The sucking reflex not present at birth

Q 11. The following are features of Trisomy 21

A. An increased incidence of glue ear
B. An increased incidence of chest infections
C. An increased risk of leukaemia
D. A decreased incidence of hypothyroidism
E. A 20% incidence of congenital heart defects

Q 12. The following conditions are inherited via X-linked recessive inheritance

A. Haemophilia A
B. Marfan syndrome
C. Duchenne muscular dystrophy
D. Noonan syndrome
E. Otosclerosis

Q 13. The following features and conditions are associated

A. Atrioventricular septal defect – Down's syndrome
B. Single palmar crease – Down's syndrome
C. Ovarian dysgenesis – Down's syndrome
D. Gynaecomastia – Klinefelter's syndrome
E. Short webbed neck – Noonan syndrome

Q 14. Regarding inherited conditions

A. Pyloric stenosis is inherited in multifactorial fashion
B. Spina bifida is of autosomal recessive inheritance with incomplete penetrance
C. Maternal diabetes mellitus is associated with sacral agenesis
D. Maternal diabetes mellitus is associated with organomegaly
E. Galactosaemia is inherited by X-linked recessive inheritance

Q 15. Visual impairment may present with the following

A. Failure to smile responsively by 6 weeks
B. Photophobia
C. Nystagmus
D. Squint
E. A white pupillary reflex

Q 16. Amblyopia

A. Usually affects both eyes
B. Is important to treat before age 7 years
C. Is a convergent squint
D. May result from refractive errors in the eye
E. May result from a capillary haemangioma obstructing the visual axis

Q 17. Physiological anisocoria

A. Is a heterogeneity of pupillary colour
B. Is a difference in pupillary size
C. Is of autosomal dominant inheritance
D. Can progress to blindness
E. Is more common in boys

Q 18. In haemophilia A

A. Spontaneous bleeding into joints does not occur in moderate disease
B. Factor VIII is necessary before surgery
C. The child should be advised that they can participate in contact sports
D. Factor VIII antibodies are rare
E. Carrier females can be detected antenatally using DNA analysis

Q 19. Beta-thalassaemia major

A. Results in a mild microcytic anaemia
B. Is a cause of splenomegaly
C. May be treated with bone marrow transplant
D. Causes painful crises
E. Can present with digital infarcts

Q 20. The following are causes of nappy rash

A. Candida infection
B. Seborrheic dermatitis
C. Atopic dermatitis
D. Psoriasis
E. Irritant dermatitis

Q 21. The following can cause blistering skin disease in children

- **A.** Coxsackie A infection
- **B.** Human herpes virus 6
- **C.** Impetigo
- **D.** Erythema multiforme
- **E.** Staphylococcal scalded skin syndrome

Q 22. Molluscum contagiosum

- **A.** Is caused by an adenovirus
- **B.** Presents as red umbilicated papules
- **C.** Contains live virus within the papules
- **D.** Usually resolves spontaneously within 8 weeks
- **E.** Should be treated with cryotherapy

Q 23. Infantile haemangiomas

- **A.** Remain present throughout life
- **B.** Are usually treated with a pulsed dye laser
- **C.** Are seen in 1 in 10 babies
- **D.** Are usually present at birth
- **E.** May be blue or red

Q 24. Phenylketonuria

- **A.** Is managed by eliminating breast milk
- **B.** Results in fair hair and skin and blue eyes in all affected children
- **C.** Is diagnosed on the Guthrie test
- **D.** Causes cataracts
- **E.** Is an autosomal dominant condition

Q 25. Anorexia nervosa

- **A.** Is more common than bulimia
- **B.** Can have a low T4 in the presence of a normal T3
- **C.** Can demonstrate a raised growth hormone
- **D.** May have a hypochloraemic hypokalaemic alkalosis
- **E.** Is associated with diarrhoea more commonly than constipation

Q 26. In the treatment of gastro-oesophageal reflux

A. A CT head scan should normally be done before a fundoplication is considered
B. Omeprazole's action is on the H1 receptors in oxyntic cells
C. A Nissen fundoplication involves a 75% wrap of the gastric fundus around the distal oesophagus
D. Positioning the infant prone at a 30 degree head-up angle is the most desirable
E. Removal of dairy produce from the diet of a breast-feeding mother will not be helpful

Q 27. Human breast milk compared to cow's milk

A. Has a higher protein content
B. Has a lower casein:whey ratio
C. Has a higher carbohydrate content
D. Has a higher calcium content
E. Has a higher iron content

Q 28. Regarding an ostium secundum atrial septal defect

A. Cardiac failure is common in infancy
B. They are commonly asymptomatic in children
C. It is the most common form of atrial septal defect
D. A pansystolic murmur is heard
E. Surgical repair is always required

Q 29. Coarctation of the aorta

A. Is associated with Turner syndrome
B. Is more common in girls
C. May present in a school age child
D. Is associated with other cardiac defects
E. May recur after surgical repair

Q 30. A ventricular septal defect is the most likely diagnosis in a 4-year-old girl who on examination has

A. An ejection systolic murmur between the shoulder blades
B. An ejection systolic murmur
C. A loud pansystolic murmur at the lower left sternal edge
D. Central cyanosis
E. A soft continous murmur that disappears on lying down

Q 31. Regarding collection of urine from children

- **A.** In an infant, two clean catch specimens are ideally required prior to treatment
- **B.** A suprapubic aspirate is the gold standard sample in sick infants under 1 year
- **C.** Contamination is a problem with bag collections
- **D.** A mid-stream urine sample can be collected from children over age 2 years
- **E.** A bag urine is preferable to a clean catch specimen in an infant

Q 32. The following are true regarding undescended testes

- **A.** Less than 1% of male infants have undescended testes at birth
- **B.** After 9 months of age undescended testes rarely descend spontaneously
- **C.** Orchidopexy increases fertility
- **D.** Orchidopexy deceases malignancy rate in the testis
- **E.** Retractile testes require surgical fixation

Q 33. Oligoarticular juvenile idiopathic arthritis

- **A.** Typically involves early morning joint stiffness
- **B.** In young children is more common in boys
- **C.** Is associated with chronic iridocyclitis in one-third of cases
- **D.** Is rheumatoid factor positive
- **E.** Typically affects the knees, ankles and elbows

Q 34. The following tend to cause an acute monoarthritis

- **A.** Perthes disease
- **B.** Haemophilia
- **C.** Kawasaki disease
- **D.** Systemic lupus erythematosis
- **E.** Inflammatory bowel disease

Q 35. Kawasaki disease

- **A.** Requires a fever for more than 3 days for the diagnosis
- **B.** May cause a bright red tongue
- **C.** If untreated has a 30% rate of coronary artery aneurysms

D. May cause myocarditis

E. Is treated with paracetamol for 6 weeks

Q 36. Regarding posture in toddlers

A. Flat feet are normal

B. Out-toeing is unusual

C. In-toeing may be due to flat feet

D. Toe-walking can affect the Achilles tendon

E. Bow legs can be normal

Q 37. Talipes

A. Calcaneovalgus is the most common form

B. If positional, requires only physiotherapy

C. Is associated with oligohydramnios

D. If equinovarus, usually requires surgery

E. Is seen in Down's syndrome

Q 38. The following are causes of sensorineural deafness in infants

A. Pierre-Robin syndrome

B. Glue ear

C. Gentamicin

D. Craniofacial malformations

E. Ear wax

Q 39. Croup

A. Is the most common cause of acute stridor in children

B. Is caused by parainfluenza virus

C. Is worse in the morning

D. Is most common in infants under 1 year of age

E. Is characterized by a severely unwell child

Q 40. Chronic nasal stuffiness can be caused by

A. Hyperthyroidism

B. Diabetes mellitus

C. Reflux

D. Sinusitis

E. Deviated nasal septum

Q 41. Regarding attention deficit hyperactivity disorder

A. The clinical features should be present for at least 6 months for the diagnosis

B. It is equally prevalent in girls as in boys

C. Stimulants make it worse

D. There is an increased risk of anxiety

E. Methylphenidate is an effective therapy

Q 42. Regarding bowel control

A. It is normally achieved by age 1.5 years

B. It is achieved more quickly in girls

C. Daytime soiling is seen in 5% of 5- to 12-year-olds

D. Faecal soiling may be caused by constipation

E. Faecal soiling is usually a sign of severe emotional disturbance

Q 43. Anxiety-related school refusal

A. Is more common in boys

B. Is associated with good school performance

C. Is associated with laziness

D. Is associated with stealing

E. May be managed with stimulants

Q 44. During pregnancy, the following substances can transmit the corresponding diseases

A. Non-pasteurized cheeses – Toxoplasmosis

B. Pâté – *Listeria monocytogenes*

C. Smoked meats – Toxoplasmosis

D. Raw eggs – *Listeria monocytogenes*

E. Cat litter – Cytomegalovirus

Q 45. Chorionic villous sampling

A. Is performed at 11 weeks' gestation

B. Samples fetal cells in the amniotic fluid

C. Has a 1% procedure-related risk of miscarriage

D. Enables diagnosis of congenital infection

E. Enables enzyme analysis for inborn errors of metabolism

Q 46. Neonatal jitteriness

    A. Is associated with apnoea
    B. May be caused by sepsis
    C. May be caused by hypocalcaemia
    D. May occur while the infant is sleeping
    E. Is associated with altered eye movements

Q 47. The following maternal disorders can cause problems in the fetus

    A. Lupus erythematosis
    B. Myasthenia gravis
    C. Hyperthyroidism
    D. Autoimmune thrombocytopenia
    E. Diabetes mellitus

Q 48. *Listeria monocytogenes* infection during pregnancy

    A. May be acquired from uncooked meats
    B. May be acquired from raw vegetables
    C. May be acquired by ascending infection from the mother
    D. May cause hydrocephalus in the infant
    E. Causes a maternal flu-like illness

Q 49. In a 1-week-old infant, the following would be abnormal

    A. Inguinal lymphadenopathy
    B. Difficulty with mouth breathing
    C. Some milk secretion from the breasts
    D. A positive Moro reflex
    E. A positive forward parachute reflex

Q 50. Clinical features of hypocalcaemia in childhood include

    A. Hypertension
    B. Peptic ulcers
    C. Papilloedema
    D. Seizures
    E. Cataracts

Q 51. Regarding type 1 diabetes mellitus

    A. The Dawn phenomenon refers to rebound hyperglycaemia at 5:00–8:00 a.m. following nocturnal hypoglycaemia

B. The Somogyi phenomenon is hypoglycaemia occurring soon after insulin therapy is commenced due to a resurgence of pancreatic β-cell activity

C. The honeymoon period usually begins 2 months after initiation of insulin treatment

D. Identical twins have a 30% concordance

E. Microalbuminuria rarely develops within 5 years of diagnosis

Q 52. Primary amenorrhoea

A. Is defined as no onset of menses by 16 years, or within 3 years of onset of secondary sexual characteristics or within 1 year of Tanner stage 5

B. May be due to McCune-Albright syndrome

C. May be due to Turner syndrome

D. May be due to polycystic ovary syndrome

E. Is always associated with secondary sexual characteristics

Q 53. A growth rate of 3 cm per year

A. Is normal in a 7-year-old boy

B. Is low in a 7-year-old girl

C. Is normal in a 14-year-old prepubertal boy

D. Is normal in a 14-year-old girl who has had the menarche

E. Is always pathological

Q 54. Children receiving long-term systemic corticosteroids

A. May develop Cushing's disease

B. Are at risk of severe chicken pox

C. Develop adrenal atrophy which may persist for years after stopping steroids

D. May present with advanced tuberculosis with relatively few symptoms

E. Are at risk of hypoglycaemia

Q 55. Erythromycin

A. Is an aminoglycoside antibiotic

B. Is active against *Haemophilus influenzae*

C. Is always effective against *Streptococcus pneumoniae*

D. Can cause urticaria

E. Is excreted in breast milk in large amounts

Q 56. Parvovirus B19

A. Is transmitted via the respiratory route
B. Causes exanthem subitum
C. Is most commonly seen in toddlers
D. Is most commonly seen during the winter
E. Can cause aplastic crises in children with sickle cell anaemia

Q 57. Hand, foot and mouth disease

A. May be spread via the faecal-oral route
B. Is most common in school age children
C. Causes vesicles in the mouth
D. Causes a generalized maculopapular rash
E. Is due to infection with adenovirus

Q 58. Regarding cat scratch disease

A. It is a viral infection seen worldwide
B. It is particularly seen secondary to scratches from kittens
C. No history of scratch is obtained in 75% of cases
D. The inoculation papule may last for months
E. It may result from a dog scratch

Q 59. The following are true of measles infection

A. The infection is transmitted via the faecal-oral route
B. The incubation period is 14–21 days
C. The typical rash appears around day 7 of the illness
D. Children are infectious until 4–5 days after the appearance of the rash
E. The infection is minimally contagious

Q 60. Chicken pox infection

A. Usually manifests a coryzal prodrome in infants
B. Can cause congenital malformations if contracted during pregnancy
C. May cause pruritis ani
D. Commonly causes oral ulceration
E. May be severe in children with atopic eczema

Q 61. The following are contraindications to childhood vaccination

A. Contact with an infectious disease
B. Family history of inflammatory bowel disease
C. Treatment with antibiotics
D. Family history of adverse reactions following vaccination
E. Prematurity

Q 62. Regarding oral poliomyelitis vaccination

A. It is a live virus
B. It should not be given if there is an immunosuppressed household contact
C. An un-immunized grandparent who cares for the child should be given the vaccine the previous week
D. It is important for carers of a recently immunized baby to wash their hands after nappy changes
E. It can be given to children who have been receiving high dose steroids in the previous 3 months

Q 63. An immunosuppressed child should not be given

A. Typhoid vaccine
B. Influenza vaccine
C. Oral polio vaccine
D. Varicella zoster vaccine
E. Rubella vaccine

Q 64. The following are live vaccines

A. Varicella zoster virus
B. Pertussis
C. Tetanus
D. Mumps
E. Rubella

Q 65. *Mycoplasma pneumoniae* infection

A. Is a cause of persistent cough
B. Has a 5- to 7-day incubation period
C. Causes a lymphopenia
D. Causes thrombocytopenia
E. Is a cause of diarrhoea

A 1.   **A.** true   **B.** true   **C.** true   **D.** false   **E.** false

The mouth should be checked to look for dental caries which may result in headaches. Concerning features in the history include an increase in severity or frequency of the headaches, behavioural changes and developmental deterioration. Abdominal pain may be related to stress and non-organic headaches.

A 2.   **A.** true   **B.** false   **C.** false   **D.** false   **E.** false

Febrile convulsions classically occur during a period of rapid temperature rise, are more common in boys and have a positive family history in around one-third of cases. Policies vary but a typical febrile convulsion in a child who has had them before in whom there are no concerns regarding the underlying infection does not need admission. The parents should be instructed to return with the child if the clinical situation changes however.

A 3.   **A.** true   **B.** false   **C.** true   **D.** false   **E.** true

Cerebral palsy is most commonly due to antenatal causes, and birth asphyxia accounts for an estimated 10% of cases in the UK. There are three types: spastic, ataxic and dyskinetic.

A 4.   **A.** false   **B.** true   **C.** false   **D.** true   **E.** true

An aura suggests a focal origin. Generalized tonic-clonic seizures are by definition always associated with loss of conciousness.

A 5.   **A.** false   **B.** true   **C.** true   **D.** false   **E.** true

There are four main areas of development: gross motor, fine motor, communication and social/emotional development. On average, girls achieve bladder control considerably earlier than boys.

A 6. **A.** true **B.** true **C.** true **D.** false **E.** false

Scribbling is attained by 15 months of age, and building a 3-cube tower by 18 months.

A 7. **A.** false **B.** false **C.** true **D.** true **E.** true

Drawing a circle and jumping are usually attained by 3 years of age.

A 8. **A.** false **B.** true **C.** true **D.** true **E.** false

Drawing a triangle and riding a bicycle are attained by 5 years of age.

A 9. **A.** false **B.** true **C.** true **D.** false **E.** true

The lateral propping reflex appears around 7 months and the forward parachute at 5–6 months.

A 10. **A.** false **B.** true **C.** false **D.** true **E.** true

The pincer grasp develops by around 9–14 months. The Landau reflex appears at 3–6 months.

A 11. **A.** true **B.** true **C.** true **D.** false **E.** false

Down's syndrome infants have an increased incidence of hypothyroidism, and around a 40% incidence of congenital heart defects.

A 12. **A.** true **B.** false **C.** true **D.** false **E.** false

Marfan syndrome, Noonan syndrome and otosclerosis are all autosomal dominant disorders.

A 13. **A.** true **B.** true **C.** false **D.** true **E.** true

Ovarian dysgenesis is seen in Turner syndrome (as is also a short webbed neck).

A 14. **A.** true **B.** false **C.** true **D.** true **E.** false

Galactosaemia is inherited via autosomal recessive inheritance.

A 15. **A.** true **B.** true **C.** true **D.** true **E.** true

A **16.** **A.** false **B.** true **C.** false **D.** true **E.** true

Amblyopia is the permanent impairment of visual acuity in an eye that has not received a clear image while vision is developing. It usually affects only one eye (a 'lazy' eye).

A **17.** **A.** false **B.** true **C.** false **D.** false **E.** false

Physiological anisocoria (a difference in pupillary size) is very common, affecting up to one-fifth of individuals to a varying degree.

A **18.** **A.** false **B.** true **C.** false **D.** false **E.** true

Spontaneous bleeding into joints occasionally occurs in moderate disease. Contact sports should be avoided. Factor VIII antibodies are seen in 10% of children.

A **19.** **A.** false **B.** true **C.** true **D.** false **E.** false

Beta-thalassaemia major causes a severe microcytic hypochromic anaemia. Painful crises and digital infarcts are seen in sickle cell anaemia.

A **20.** **A.** true **B.** true **C.** true **D.** true **E.** true

A **21.** **A.** true **B.** false **C.** true **D.** true **E.** true

Coxsackie A infection causes hand, foot and mouth disease in which there are vesicles on the palms, soles and mouth. Particular forms of staphylococcal infection cause bullous impetigo and staphylococcal scalded skin syndrome (which may begin with blisters). Erythema multiforme may rarely be bullous. HHV-6 causes slapped cheek disease which does not involve blistering.

A **22.** **A.** false **B.** false **C.** true **D.** false **E.** false

Molluscum contagiosum is caused by a pox virus. The papules are flesh-coloured and umbilicated. Spontaneous resolution is the usual course, but may take several months. Treatment with cryotherapy can be done but is painful, and usually not necessary.

A 23. A. false **B.** false **C.** false **D.** false **E.** true

Infantile haemangiomas are benign vascular tumours which enlarge during the first 6–9 months and then involute. They are present in 1 in 20 babies and usually appear during the first 3 weeks after birth. If superficial they appear red, and if deep they appear blue. No treatment is required unless they become complicated, in which case oral steroids can prevent enlargement, or surgery is used if necessary. A pulsed dye laser is used to treat ulcerated lesions.

A 24. A. false **B.** false **C.** true **D.** false **E.** false

Phenylketonuria is an autosomal recessive condition. It is managed by excluding phenylalanine from the diet. If a strict diet is adhered to the classical phenotype does not occur.

A 25. A. false **B.** false **C.** true **D.** true **E.** false

T3 is more often low with an apparently normal T4. Diarrhoea may occur with laxative abuse but constipation is more common with inherent hypomobility of the gut.

A 26. A. false **B.** false **C.** false **D.** false **E.** false

Omeprazole (licensed down to 2 years of age) affects the proton pump in the parietal cell by binding irreversibly to it. A Thal fundoplication is a 75% wraparound whereas a Nissen is a total wraparound. The left lateral position decreases GOR, but prone is contraindicated due to SIDS association. It is clear that small amounts of cow's milk protein passing through the breast milk are sufficient to cause vomiting due to an allergy or intolerance to cow's milk.

Thomson M. Disorders of the oesaphagus and stomach in infants. *Bailliere's Clin Gastroenterol* 1997; **11**(3): 547–71.

A 27. A. false **B.** true **C.** true **D.** false **E.** true

Human breast milk is very different from cow's milk. It contains much less protein and lower calcium and phosphate levels. The fat levels are slightly higher in human breast milk. The carbohydrate content is much higher in human breast milk, and there is a much lower casein:whey ratio.

28. **A.** false **B.** true **C.** true **D.** false **E.** false

With an ostium secundum ASD cardiac failure is unusual until adult life. The murmur is an ejection systolic murmur at the upper left sternal edge. Small defects will usually close spontaneously.

29. **A.** true **B.** false **C.** true **D.** true **E.** true

Coarctation of the aorta may present late on a routine check with an asymptomatic murmur and/or hypertension in the upper limbs and weak peripheral pulses. It may also present late symptomatically with heart failure. Recurrence rates after repair are approximately 30%.

30. **A.** false **B.** false **C.** true **D.** false **E.** false

A ventricular septal defect has a loud pansystolic murmur at the lower left sternal edge. Smaller holes have shorter and louder murmurs. There may be a parasternal thrill felt. There is a loud second heart sound if pulmonary hypertension is present.

31. **A.** false **B.** true **C.** true **D.** false **E.** false

A clean catch specimen is preferable to a bag urine specimen in an infant as contamination is less of a problem. Mid-stream urine samples can generally be obtained from children over 3 years.

32. **A.** false **B.** true **C.** true **D.** false **E.** false

Approximately 3.5% of boys have undescended testes at birth. Orchidopexy does not reduce the incidence of malignant transformation (which is increased in undescended testes), however it allows earlier detection of malignancy, and therefore treatment.

33. **A.** true **B.** false **C.** true **D.** false **E.** true

Oligoarticular juvenile idiopathic arthritis is more common in girls below the age of 4 years. Those who are ANA positive are at greater risk of eye disease. Rheumatoid factor and HLA-B27 are negative.

34. **A.** true **B.** true **C.** false **D.** false **E.** false

Kawasaki disease, SLE and inflammatory bowel disease tend to cause a polyarthritis. Haemophilia can result in either a poly- or monoarthritis.

Exam 3

Answers

A **35.** **A.** false **B.** true **C.** false **D.** true **E.** false

The diagnostic criteria for Kawasaki disease are a fever above 38.5 °C for greater then 5 days, and four of the following: bilateral non-purulent conjunctivitis, oral mucosal changes including a bright red tongue, cervical adenopathy with one node greater than 1.5 cm, swollen hands and feet and a polymorphous rash. 20–40% of untreated children develop coronary artery aneurysms.

A **36.** **A.** true **B.** false **C.** true **D.** true **E.** true

Toddlers have flat feet due to ligamentous laxity and a fat pad under the foot. Out-toeing and bow legs are both common and usually normal in toddlers, though bow legs may be pathological (e.g. rickets, Blount's disease).

A **37.** **A.** false **B.** true **C.** true **D.** false **E.** false

Talipes is a positional deformity of the foot. Talipes equinovarus is the most common form in which the foot is supinated with the heel inwardly rotated and the forefoot adducted. This may be positional, in which case it will correct to the normal anatomical position during examination and requires only physiotherapy. Fixed talipes requires intervention by either conservative (using serial plasters) or surgical means.

A **38.** **A.** false **B.** false **C.** true **D.** true **E.** false

Pierre-Robin syndrome, glue ear and ear wax all cause conductive deafness. Craniofacial malformations can cause both conductive and sensorineural deafness.

A **39.** **A.** true **B.** true **C.** false **D.** false **E.** false

Croup is caused by a viral infection, commonly parainfluenza, occasionally respiratory syncytial virus. It is worse in the evenings and at night. It is classically seen in infants aged 1–2 years, and the child is not usually particularly unwell, unlike epiglottitis in which the child is severely unwell.

A **40.** **A.** false **B.** true **C.** true **D.** true **E.** true

Hypothyroidism can cause nasal stuffiness.

A. true **B.** false **C.** false **D.** true **E.** true

Attention deficit hyperactivity disorder (ADHD) is characterized by inattention, hyperactivity and impulsivity. These features should be present for at least 6 months, and commence below age 7 years. They should also occur in more than one setting, and cause significant social or school impairment. It is more common in boys. There is an associated risk of anxiety, conduct disorder and aggression. Both methylphenidate and amphetamines are effective treatments.

A 42. **A.** false **B.** true **C.** false **D.** true **E.** false

Bowel control is normally achieved by age 2 years, though there is wide variation. Daytime soiling is seen in only 1–2% of 5- to 12-year-olds. Faecal soiling is involuntary and may be due to organic causes (faecal retention with overflow incontinence or neurological damage) or be secondary to stress. Encopresis is the voluntary passage of faeces in abnormal places in an otherwise healthy child beyond the usual age for toilet training, is due to non-organic causes and can be a sign of severe emotional distress.

A 43. **A.** false **B.** true **C.** false **D.** false **E.** false

Anxiety-related school refusal is more common in girls. It is associated with insecurity and separation anxiety from parents, and with good school performance. Truancy is more common in boys and is associated with laziness, poor motivation and antisocial behaviour (e.g. stealing). Management is psychotherapy based.

A 44. **A.** false **B.** true **C.** true **D.** false **E.** false

Listeria monocytogenes can be transmitted by non-pasteurized products and soft cheeses, pâté, raw vegetables and warmed pre-cooked meats. Toxoplasmosis can be transmitted via uncooked meats and smoked meats, raw eggs and unwashed fruits and vegetables.

A 45. **A.** true **B.** false **C.** true **D.** true **E.** true

Chorionic villous sampling may be done from 11–14 weeks' gestation. There is a 1% procedure-related risk (and overall 3–4% risk) of miscarriage. It allows chromosome analysis earlier than

Exam 3

Answers

amniocentesis and other rarer mutations can also be screened for. Major trisomies and sex chromosome aneuploidies can be diagnosed. Also enzyme analysis for certain inborn errors of metabolism and congenital infection, using PCR to detect viral particle DNA, can be carried out.

A **46.** **A.** false **B.** true **C.** true **D.** true **E.** false

Neonatal jitteriness is characterized by rhythmic movements that may occur while the infant is awake or while they are asleep, and there are no altered eye movements associated (unlike neonatal seizures, with which they can be confused). Neonatal jitteriness may be caused by hypoglycaemia, hypocalcaemia and sepsis.

A **47.** **A.** true **B.** true **C.** true **D.** true **E.** true

They can all cause problems in the fetus. Lupus erythematosis, myasthenia gravis, hyperthyroidism and autoimmune thrombocytopenia all exert their effect via placental antibody transfer. Maternal diabetes mellitus is associated with several fetal malformations and neonatal hypoglycaemia.

A **48.** **A.** true **B.** true **C.** true **D.** true **E.** true

Listeria monocytogenes infection may be acquired from various foods, including unpasteurized milk products, especially soft cheeses, but also raw vegetables and uncooked meats. It may be caused by transplacental infection or an ascending infection. There are various different effects it may have on the fetus including premature delivery, abortion or stillbirth, pneumonia, sepsis and disseminated infection with seizures, rash and hepatosplenomegaly. Hydrocephalus is a relatively common sequelae.

A **49.** **A.** false **B.** false **C.** false **D.** false **E.** true

The forward parachute reflex appears at 5–6 months and remains for life. Inguinal and cervical lymphadenopathy is present in around a third of newborns, and should not be considered pathological on its own.

Bamji M, Stone RK, Kaul A *et al*. Palpable lymph nodes in healthy newborns and infants. *Pediatrics* 1986; **78**: 573–5.

A. false **B.** false **C.** true **D.** true **E.** true

Clinical features of hypocalcaemia include muscle cramps, paraesthesia, seizures, laryngeal and carpopedal spasm and tetany, cataracts and soft teeth. Both hypertension and peptic ulcers are features of hypercalcaemia.

A 51. **A.** false **B.** false **C.** false **D.** false **E.** false

The 'Somogyi phenomenon' is rebound hyperglycaemia following hypoglycaemia. It should be suspected if high morning blood glucoses are occurring, when it reflects hypoglycaemia during the night, and so blood glucose should be checked at 2:00–3:00 a.m. The 'Dawn phenomenon' refers to a rise in blood glucose that occurs in the early morning (5:00–8:00 a.m). This is thought to be due to a combination of factors including the increase in cortisol level, the effect of increased nocturnal growth hormone and low insulin levels due to the length of time after the evening dose. The 'honeymoon' period usually begins 1–2 weeks after initiation of insulin treatment and lasts for a variable period of time. It is a time of minimal or falling insulin requirements due to residual endogenous insulin production. Identical twins have over 50% concordance for type 1 diabetes mellitus. Microalbuminuria tends to develop after 10–15 years of diagnosis.

A 52. **A.** true **B.** false **C.** true **D.** true **E.** false

McCune-Albright syndrome comprises precocious puberty and polyostotic fibrous dysplasia. There may be multiple hormonal overactivity seen.

A 53. **A.** false **B.** true **C.** true **D.** true **E.** false

A normal 7-year-old child has a growth rate of 5–6 cm per year. A prepubertal 14-year-old boy is awaiting his pubertal growth spurt, and a 14-year-old girl who has had the menarche can have had her growth spurt.

A 54. **A.** false **B.** true **C.** true **D.** true **E.** false

Children on long-term systemic corticosteroids can develop Cushing's syndrome (moon face, striae, acne). Cushing's disease refers to Cushing's syndrome secondary to a pituitary tumour. Other side-effects are hyperglycaemia and immunosuppression,

Exam 3

Answers

and atypical clinical presentations of infections, such that infections may reach an advanced stage before being recognized. A particular risk is chicken pox which can be severe, and passive immunization with varicella zoster immunoglobulin (VZIG) should be given to exposed children.

A 55. **A.** false   **B.** false   **C.** false   **D.** true   **E.** false

Erythromycin is a macrolide antibiotic. It has a spectrum of activity similar to penicillin. It has poor activity against *Haemophilus influenzae*, and there are resistant strains of *Streptococcus pneumoniae*. Only small amounts of erythromycin are excreted in breast milk.

A 56. **A.** true   **B.** false   **C.** false   **D.** false   **E.** true

Parvovirus B19 causes slapped cheek disease, which is most commonly seen in school age children during the spring. Children with chronic haemolysis including those with sickle cell anaemia and thalassaemia can get a transient aplastic crisis as the virus attacks the red cell precursors leading to a transient arrest of erythropoiesis. Exanthem subitum is also known as Roseola infantum and is caused by herpes virus 6.

A 57. **A.** true   **B.** false   **C.** true   **D.** true   **E.** false

Hand, foot and mouth disease is due to enteroviral infection including Coxsackie A or B. It may be spread via the faecal-oral or droplet route, or by direct contact. The disease is usually seen in preschool children. It causes a mild illness with fever, vesicles in the mouth, palms and soles, and a generalized maculopapular rash, particularly with papules on the buttocks.

A 58. **A.** false   **B.** false   **C.** false   **D.** true   **E.** true

Cat scratch disease is due to a bacterial infection with *Bartonella henselae*. In around half of cases no history of scratch is obtained. In half of cases an inoculation papule or pustule is present which may last from days to months. Conjunctivitis and regional lymphadenopathy are also seen.

A 59. **A.** false   **B.** false   **C.** false   **D.** true   **E.** false

Measles is spread by droplet infection. The incubation period is 7–14 days, and the rash appears around day 2–3 of the illness.

A 60. A. false **B.** true **C.** true **D.** true **E.** true

Chicken pox infection often has no prodrome in young infants. If contracted during pregnancy during the first or second trimesters, it can rarely cause congenital varicella syndrome involving zig-zag scarring of the skin, limb malformations, and CNS and eye defects.

A 61. A. false **B.** false **C.** false **D.** false **E.** false

None of these conditions are contraindications to childhood vaccination.

A 62. A. true **B.** true **C.** false **D.** true **E.** false

The oral polio vaccine is a live virus and therefore should not be given to an immunosuppressed child including one who has received high dose steroids in the previous 3 months. The virus is secreted in the stools and therefore it is important for carers to wash their hands carefully when changing the nappy, and for an un-immunized grandparent who cares for the child to be given the vaccine at the same time. In addition, it should not be given if there is an immunosuppressed contact in the household.

A 63. A. false **B.** false **C.** true **D.** true **E.** true

Immunosuppressed children should not be given live vaccines. These include measles, mumps, rubella, oral polio, varicella zoster virus and yellow fever vaccines.

A 64. A. true **B.** false **C.** false **D.** true **E.** true

Pertussis is a killed organism vaccine and tetanus is a toxoid vaccine.

A 65. A. true **B.** false **C.** false **D.** false **E.** true

Mycoplasma pneumoniae has a 10- to 14-day incubation period. The most frequent presentation is with bronchopneumonia in school age children. It produces cold agglutinins which cause a haemolytic anaemia. There are many other clinical features including rashes, myalgia and arthralgia, vomiting, diarrhoea and hepatitis and encephalitis.

Q 1. Acute cerebellar ataxia may be secondary to

A. Heavy metal poisoning
B. Midline cerebellar haemorrhage
C. Varicella infection
D. Maple syrup urine disease
E. Phenytoin therapy

Q 2. The following can cause toe-walking in toddlers

A. Spastic diplegic cerebral palsy
B. Muscular dystrophy
C. Normal development
D. Congenital shortening of the Achilles tendon
E. Spinal dysraphism

Q 3. The following are features of a craniopharyngioma

A. It is an infratentorial tumour
B. It causes diabetes mellitus
C. It is a cause of hydrocephalus
D. It is visible on plain X-ray in half of cases
E. It is a cause of short stature

Q 4. Tics are associated with

A. Down's syndrome
B. Autism
C. Amphetamines
D. Fragile X syndrome
E. Post-rubella syndrome

Q 5. A 10-month-old child who is developing normally will

A. Scribble
B. Transfer objects from hand to hand
C. Have a pincer grasp

D. Have a palmar grasp

E. Sit well unsupported

Q 6. The majority of normal children aged 2 years can

A. Build a bridge with 3 cubes

B. Undress

C. Dress

D. Do symbolic play

E. Jump

Q 7. Walking in infancy

A. Is achieved later in boys

B. Is achieved by age 14 months in all normal children

C. Commences earlier in bottom-shufflers

D. May be achieved by age 11 months

E. Is delayed in breech babies

Q 8. At 6 months of age the following primitive reflexes are normally present

A. The Moro reflex

B. The Landau reflex

C. The palmar grasp

D. The rooting reflex

E. The stepping reflex

Q 9. A normal healthy child will acquire the following skills by the ages stated

A. Draw a square – 4 years

B. Draw a cross – 3 years

C. Say 5 words – 1 year

D. Feed with a spoon – 1 year

E. Eat using fingers – 6 months

Q 10. The following findings are suggestive of abnormal development

A. Pincer grasp not achieved by age 11 months

B. Hand preference by age 11 months

C. Head lag while held prone present at 6 weeks

D. Not babbling by 6 months of age

E. Sitting with a bent back at 6 months

Q 11. The following tests are done at the specified gestation

    A. Amniocentesis – 11 weeks
    B. Fetal anomaly ultrasound scan – 25 weeks
    C. Percutaneous umbilical blood sampling – after 17 weeks
    D. Chorionic villous sampling – 7 weeks
    E. Nuchal ultrasound scan – 12 weeks

Q 12. Regarding X-linked recessive disorders

    A. Female carriers are always affected mildly
    B. There is no transmission from father to son
    C. Daughters of affected males will always be carriers
    D. They include G6PD deficiency
    E. They include galactosaemia

Q 13. The following are features of fetal alcohol syndrome

    A. Cleft palate
    B. Single palmar crease
    C. Microcephaly
    D. Long philtrum
    E. Hypoplastic nails

Q 14. Maternal diabetes mellitus can cause

    A. Nasal hypoplasia
    B. Organomegaly
    C. Neural tube defects
    D. Sacral agenesis
    E. Transient neonatal hyperglycaemia

Q 15. Regarding neonatal conjunctivitis

    A. It is not usually purulent
    B. Gonococcal infection presents after the first week of life
    C. Chlamydia infection usually presents within hours of birth
    D. It usually requires oral antibiotic therapy
    E. If due to gonococcal infection, it is treated with fusidic acid

Q 16. In congenital glaucoma

    A. The red reflex is absent
    B. Photophobia is not present

C. It is usually unilateral

D. The eyes tend to become hypermetropic

E. It is seen in 1 in 30 000 births

Q 17. Regarding infantile convergent squint

A. It is the most common type of squint

B. It develops between 1 and 2 years of age

C. It is associated with myopia

D. Treatment is with eye patching

E. Corrective surgery is usually required

Q 18. Twin-twin transfusion syndrome

A. Does not occur in dichorionic twins

B. Is most dangerous for the plethoric twin

C. Can cause preterm delivery

D. If untreated has a very high mortality for the twins

E. If treated in utero has a low mortality for the twins

Q 19. Hyposplenism can be caused by

A. Chronic lymphocytic leukaemia

B. Bacterial endocarditis

C. Sickle cell anaemia

D. Crohn's disease

E. Beta-thalassaemia major

Q 20. Features of tuberous sclerosis include

A. Facial angiofibromas from birth

B. Café-au-lait macules

C. Infantile spasms

D. Autism

E. Lisch nodules

Q 21. Psoriasis in children

A. May be triggered by a sore throat

B. Can present with intractable nappy rash

C. Is often complicated by juvenile psoriatic arthritis

D. Usually requires treatment with phototherapy

E. Often involves pitting of the nails

Q 22. Eczema herpeticum

A. Is eczema secondary to infection with herpes simplex virus
B. Should be treated with aciclovir if severe
C. May cause fever and malaise
D. Is rarely complicated by secondary bacterial infection
E. Cannot recur severely

Q 23. Vitiligo

A. Is associated with halo naevi
B. If segmental has a worse prognosis
C. Is associated with Turner syndrome
D. Is usually asymmetrical
E. Rarely has a positive family history

Q 24. In Wilson's disease

A. Aplastic anaemia is a feature
B. There are increased copper levels in many tissues
C. Cirrhosis is a feature
D. Screening of relatives is not possible
E. It is a glycogen storage disorder

Q 25. With *Helicobacter pylori* in children

A. Positive serology indicates active infection
B. Failure to thrive is associated in developing countries
C. Intrafamilial spread is the likely cause of reinfection
D. Hyperacidic host response is likely to lead to development of gastric adenocarcinoma
E. Therapy with one antibiotic and a PPI is considered ideal

Q 26. Hepatitis A

A. Is infective until just after the jaundice appears
B. Can be associated with a Coombs positive haemolytic anaemia
C. Can be diagnosed by the finding on electron microscopy of viral particles in the faeces
D. Has a 10% chance of hepatocellular carcinoma in the 30 years following infection
E. Is caused by a DNA hepadnavirus

Q 27. **Features of non-organic origin of recurrent abdominal pain in children and adolescents are**

  A. Early morning wakening with pain
  B. Absence of dysuria
  C. Predominance in girls
  D. A family history of atypical migraine
  E. Negative correlation with *Helicobacter pylori* serological positivity

Q 28. **In supraventricular tachycardia**

  A. Intermittent *p* waves are present
  B. Capture beats are present
  C. It can be stimulated by a hot bath
  D. It can present with hydrops fetalis
  E. In infants, it can be stopped by immersing the face in cold water

Q 29. **The Duckett-Jones major criteria for the diagnosis of rheumatic fever include**

  A. Gottron's papules
  B. Fever
  C. Short PR interval
  D. Previous rheumatic fever
  E. Subcutaneous nodules

Q 30. **The following clinical features can be seen in infective endocarditis**

  A. Splenomegaly
  B. Arthritis of large joints
  C. Osler's nodes
  D. Erythematous rash on thenar and hypothenar eminence
  E. Haematuria

Q 31. **In the nephrotic syndrome**

  A. Oedema is rarely present
  B. Diarrhoea is a feature
  C. Frothy urine is usually present
  D. Most commonly there is a membranous nephropathy
  E. Hyperlipidaemia is occasionally seen

Q 32. The features of acute nephritic syndrome include

- **A.** Oedema
- **B.** Polyuria
- **C.** Red cell casts in the urine
- **D.** Hypertension
- **E.** Hyperkalaemia

Q 33. In infants with neonatal lupus

- **A.** Complete heart block is present in over two-thirds of cases
- **B.** It is associated with anti-Jo1 antibodies in the mother
- **C.** Most mothers have clinical SLE
- **D.** The cutaneous features continue for 1–2 years
- **E.** Subsequent pregnancies will be similarly affected

Q 34. The following infections can be associated with a vasculitis

- **A.** HIV
- **B.** Tuberculosis
- **C.** Epstein-Barr virus
- **D.** Chicken pox
- **E.** Bacterial endocarditis

Q 35. In rheumatic fever

- **A.** Polyarthralgia is a minor diagnostic criteria
- **B.** Valvular lesions take 1–2 months to develop
- **C.** The arthritis affects predominantly the small joints of the hands and feet
- **D.** The arthritis is poorly responsive to salicylates
- **E.** Individual joints usually remain inflamed for over a month

Q 36. Scheuermann's disease

- **A.** Manifests in preschool children
- **B.** Affects the cervical spine
- **C.** Is self-limiting
- **D.** Is usually painless
- **E.** Is more common in overweight boys

Q 37. Perthes disease

- **A.** Classically presents during adolescence
- **B.** Is bilateral in one-third of cases

C. Is visible in the early stages on MRI scan
D. Requires osteotomy if the child is under 5 years old
E. Causes a semi-flexed internally rotated leg at rest

Q 38. In glue ear

A. There has been fluid in the middle ear for more than 4 weeks
B. Tympanometry will show an exaggerated response
C. It is managed with an initial observation period for 6 months to allow spontaneous resolution
D. The eardrum may look normal
E. It may present with behavioural difficulties

Q 39. Recurrent (spasmodic) croup

A. Is most common in infants under 1 year
B. Is usually unresponsive to steroids
C. Is related to bronchial hyper-reactivity
D. Can result in bronchiectasis
E. Is caused by *Staphylococcus aureus*

Q 40. Bronchiolitis

A. May be due to parainfluenza viruses
B. Rarely causes apnoea
C. Is always improved with bronchodilators
D. Cannot recur
E. May be due to rhinovirus

Q 41. Recurrent abdominal pain is likely to be organic if

A. There is rectal mucus
B. The pain awakens the child at night
C. The pain is paraumbilical
D. There is dysuria
E. There is good school performance

Q 42. Toddler food refusal can be helped by

A. Ensuring the parents remain relaxed during mealtimes
B. Giving favourite foods for puddings
C. Sticking to a few foods the toddler is comfortable with
D. Having meals when the toddler asks for them
E. Ensuring the toddler finishes all on the plate at mealtimes

Q **43. Attention deficit hyperactivity disorder**

A. Has an equal sex ratio
B. May improve on a cow's milk-free diet
C. Is more likely to develop if a first-degree relative has ADHD
D. Is associated with increased incidence of criminal behaviour in adulthood
E. Is associated with epilepsy

Q **44. The antenatal nuchal scan**

A. Is performed at 10–13 weeks
B. May be used to assess cervical integrity
C. Showing an increased nuchal fold thickness is indicative of Down's syndrome with 85% sensitivity
D. Showing an increased nuchal fold thickness has a 2% false positive rate for Down's syndrome
E. Has a 92% sensitivity rate when nuchal fold thickness is combined with maternal PAPP-A and inhibin levels

Q **45. The following conditions may cause an increased maternal serum alpha-fetoprotein**

A. Incorrect gestational age dating
B. Multiple pregnancy
C. Spina bifida
D. Intrauterine growth retardation
E. Down's syndrome

Q **46. In a normal newborn**

A. It is not necessary to check for congenital dislocation of the hip if there are no associated risk factors
B. Serious cardiac pathology is always apparent by 48 hours of age
C. The Landau reflex is present
D. The Moro reflex is not always present
E. Meconium must be passed by 24 hours of age

Q **47. It is possible to test for the following disorders on the Guthrie test**

A. HIV
B. Hypothyroidism

C. Cystic fibrosis

D. Sickle cell anaemia

E. Beta-thalassaemia

Q 48. Regarding birth injuries

A. Facial nerve palsy is usually upper motor neuron damage

B. The clavicle is the most frequently fractured bone

C. In fractures of the humerus it most often involves the lower third

D. A cephalhaematoma may cause neonatal jaundice

E. Erb's palsy often follows shoulder dystocia

Q 49. Jaundice and a bilirubin level of 170 micromol/L (conjugated 80 micromol/L) in a 3-week-old baby may be due to

A. Biliary atresia

B. Neonatal hepatitis

C. Breast milk jaundice

D. G6PD deficiency

E. Severe bruising at birth

Q 50. Features of congenital hypothyroidism include

A. Umbilical hernia

B. Flat nasal bridge

C. Irritability

D. Absent posterior fontanelle

E. Feeding difficulties

Q 51. The following conditions can cause diabetes insipidus

A. Cystic fibrosis

B. Pneumonia

C. Asthma

D. Meningitis

E. Cranial radiotherapy

Q 52. Causes of tall stature during childhood include

A. Hyperthyroidism

B. Sotos syndrome

C. Marfan syndrome

D. Diabetes mellitus

E. Precocious puberty

Q 53. In normal puberty in boys

A. The first sign is appearance of pubic hair

B. The prostate enlarges

C. Facial hair appears before axillary hair

D. The sebaceous glands are stimulated by adrenal mineralocorticoids

E. Unilateral gynaecomastia may develop

Q 54. Tetracyclines

A. Can cause benign intracranial hypertension

B. Are contraindicated in children under 14 years of age

C. Are safe to use in children with renal disease

D. May cause a photosensitivity

E. Can be taken while breast-feeding

Q 55. Metronidazole

A. Is present in small amounts in breast milk

B. Commonly causes ataxia

C. May cause a darkening of the urine

D. Is always effective against Giardiasis

E. Is a cause of the red man syndrome

Q 56. Scarlet fever

A. Is due to Group B streptococcal infection

B. Features a rash which is coarse to the touch

C. Is treated with oral doxycycline

D. Produces features caused by an exotoxin

E. Is usually secondary to enteric infection

Q 57. Rubella

A. Is infectious from the onset of the rash

B. Causes a rash on the body first progressing to involve the face

C. Causes conjunctivitis

D. Is more likely to be symptomatic in younger children

E. Is usually seen during the autumn

Q 58. Infectious mononucleosis

    A. Has an incubation period of up to 2 months
    B. Can cause an arthropathy
    C. Causes a non-tender splenomegaly
    D. Infects the T lymphocytes
    E. May be reliably diagnosed using the Monospot test in young children

Q 59. Slapped cheek disease

    A. Has a 3-day incubation period
    B. May cause a remitting rash over many weeks
    C. Is spread by the faecal-oral route
    D. Can cause lymphopenia in immunocompromised children
    E. Can cause an aplasia crisis in sickle cell children

Q 60. Mumps infection

    A. Can cause problems with eating
    B. Is spread by droplet infection
    C. Is usually asymptomatic
    D. Has a 7-day incubation period
    E. Usually involves the submandibular lymph nodes

Q 61. The following are contraindications to childhood vaccination

    A. Previous history of measles
    B. Treatment with inhaled steroids
    C. Breast-feeding
    D. Recent surgery
    E. Cerebral palsy

Q 62. Whole cell pertussis vaccine

    A. Can be given to children over the age of 1 year
    B. Gives a better immunological response than acellular pertussis vaccine
    C. Is less likely to produce local side-effects in older children than acellular pertussis
    D. Can be given to a child with an evolving neurological condition
    E. Cannot be given to a child with leukaemia

Q 63. Diphtheria vaccination

    A. Is an egg protein vaccine

    B. May be given to a child receiving oral steroid therapy

    C. Cannot be given to a child having radiotherapy

    D. Contains neomycin

    E. Should not be given to a child with leukaemia

Q 64. Live vaccines cannot be given to

    A. A child with severe eczema

    B. A child who has had measles

    C. A child who has had chicken pox contact within the previous week

    D. An infant with neonatal jaundice

    E. A child with cerebral palsy

Q 65. Varicella zoster (shingles) infection

    A. If seen in infancy usually indicates defective immunocompetence

    B. Causes a very painful dermatomal rash in children

    C. Should always be treated with aciclovir

    D. May cause a facial nerve palsy

    E. Causes Ramsay Hunt syndrome

A 1.   **A.** true   **B.** true   **C.** true   **D.** true   **E.** true

The most common causes of acute ataxia in children are drugs (in particular anti-epileptics) and post-infectious cerebellitis following varicella infection. An intermittent ataxia with concurrent illness occurs in children with maple syrup urine disease.

A 2.   **A.** true   **B.** true   **C.** true   **D.** true   **E.** true

All of the above may cause toe-walking in toddlers, including as a part of normal development.

A 3.   **A.** false   **B.** false   **C.** true   **D.** false   **E.** true

Craniopharyngioma is one of the most common supratentorial tumours. It causes local pressure effects and central endocrine effects including diabetes insipidus and growth hormone deficiency causing short stature. Pressure on the optic chiasm produces temporal visual field defects though young children are often unaware of the visual loss. About 90% of tumours show calcification visible on plain X-ray.

A 4.   **A.** true   **B.** true   **C.** true   **D.** true   **E.** true

A 5.   **A.** false   **B.** true   **C.** true   **D.** true   **E.** true

Most normal children can scribble by 18 months, and do circular scribbles by 2 years.

A 6.   **A.** false   **B.** true   **C.** false   **D.** true   **E.** false

Most normal 2-year-olds can build a tower of 6 cubes. Most normal children are able to build a bridge, dress and jump by age 3 years.

A 7. **A.** false **B.** false **C.** false **D.** true **E.** false

The age at which a child walks is very variable, and can range from 11 to 15 months. Children who bottom-shuffle rather than crawl are generally late walkers, as the former is such an efficient method of transport.

A 8. **A.** false **B.** true **C.** false **D.** false **E.** false

The Moro reflex disappears at 4–5 months. The Landau reflex remains present for life. The palmar grasp disappears at 3–4 months. The rooting and stepping reflexes both disappear at 6–8 weeks.

A 9. **A.** false **B.** false **C.** false **D.** false **E.** true

Most normal children can draw a cross by 4 years and a square by 4.5 years. Most normal children can say 5–10 words and eat with a spoon by 18 months.

A 10. **A.** false **B.** true **C.** true **D.** true **E.** false

The pincer grasp can be developed from 9 to 14 months. Most infants are beginning to babble from 3 to 6 months. Marked hand preference prior to 1 year of age can be a sign of neurological damage. Infants can sit by 6 months but the back is bent: by 9 months they can sit well with a straight back.

A 11. **A.** false **B.** false **C.** false **D.** false **E.** true

Amniocentesis is done at 16–18 weeks, the fetal anomaly scan at 20 weeks, chorionic villous sampling at 11–14 weeks and percutaneous blood sampling from 20 weeks.

A 12. **A.** false **B.** true **C.** true **D.** true **E.** false

Galactosaemia is inherited by autosomal recessive inheritance.

A 13. **A.** true **B.** false **C.** true **D.** true **E.** false

The features of fetal alcohol syndrome include the facial features of a flat nasal bridge, a long philtrum, midfacial hypoplasia, upturned nose, micrognathia, ear and eye abnormalities. They also have microcephaly, developmental delay, growth retardation, and cardiac, renal and limb abnormalities.

A. false **B.** true **C.** false **D.** true **E.** false

The effects on the fetus of maternal diabetes mellitus include a large baby with organomegaly, transient neonatal hypoglycaemia, sacral agenesis, congenital heart disease and renal vein thrombosis.

A 15. **A.** false **B.** false **C.** false **D.** false **E.** false

Gonococcal infection presents within hours of birth with an extremely pussy eye and can progress to perforation within 24 hours if untreated. Treatment is with eye irrigation with crystalline penicillin and intravenous penicillin. Chlamydia infection may present after 2–3 weeks. Treatment with antibiotic eye drops is usually sufficient for the common staphylococcal infections.

A 16. **A.** false **B.** false **C.** false **D.** false **E.** false

Congenital glaucoma is usually bilateral but the eyes are unequally affected. The incidence is approximately 1 in 10 000 births. There is photophobia, and the eyes have a tendency to become myopic.

A 17. **A.** false **B.** false **C.** false **D.** false **E.** true

Infantile convergent squint usually develops during the first few months of age as an isolated phenomenon. Corrective surgery is usually required.

A 18. **A.** true **B.** true **C.** true **D.** true **E.** false

Even with treatment, survival in both twins is about 66%.

A 19. **A.** false **B.** false **C.** true **D.** false **E.** false

Bacterial endocarditis and chronic lymphocytic leukaemia cause splenomegaly.

A 20. **A.** false **B.** true **C.** true **D.** true **E.** false

Tuberous sclerosis is a relatively common inherited neurocutaneous disorder. Two gene sites have been identified (on chromosome 9 and chromosome 16). The classic triad of features is facial angiofibromas (also known as adenoma sebaceum),

Exam 4

Answers

seizures and mental retardation. Features are however very variable and less than one-third will develop the classical picture. The features progress over time, and facial angiofibromas are not usually present at birth, but generally develop by 2–5 years.

A **21.** **A.** true **B.** true **C.** false **D.** false **E.** true

Psoriasis in children (of a small plaque guttate type picture) may be triggered by Group A haemolytic Streptococcal infection. In infants, it is a cause of intractable nappy rash. Juvenile psoriatic arthritis is extremely rare, but nail pitting is seen in up to 80% of cases. Treatment with topical therapy is usually sufficient.

A **22.** **A.** false **B.** false **C.** true **D.** false **E.** false

Eczema herpeticum is herpes infection in a child with atopic eczema. It can be severe causing systemic upset and should always be treated with systemic aciclovir. Secondary bacterial infection is common. Recurrences (just as severe or worse than previous attacks) are not uncommon.

A **23.** **A.** true **B.** false **C.** false **D.** false **E.** false

Vitiligo is a disorder of depigmentation in which melanocytes are destroyed. There is a positive family history in around 40%. The depigmentation is usually roughly symmetrical. The childhood segmental form has a good prognosis.

A **24.** **A.** false **B.** true **C.** true **D.** false **E.** false

Wilson's disease is a disorder of copper transport and is inherited in autosomal recessive fashion. Relatives can and should be screened as they may have mild clinical features and require treatment.

A **25.** **A.** false **B.** true **C.** true **D.** false **E.** false

A **26.** **A.** true **B.** true **C.** true **D.** false **E.** false

Hepatitis A has no long-term sequelae, unlike B or C where the chance of subsequent hepatocellular carcinoma is 3–10% and 15% respectively. Hepatitis A is caused by an RNA picornavirus.

A 27. **A.** false **B.** false **C.** true **D.** false **E.** false

Any nocturnal wakening with pain must be investigated for an organic cause. UTIs can occur without symptoms and an MSU is necessary in the majority of children with abdominal pain even if a psychogenic origin is suspected. Abdominal migraine occurs and has a preceding family history of classical migraine. There is no correlation, positive or negative, between *Helicobacter pylori* serology and recurrent abdominal pain of non-organic or organic origin.

A 28. **A.** false **B.** false **C.** true **D.** true **E.** true

In supraventricular tachycardia (SVT) regular *p* waves are present. Capture beats are a feature of ventricular tachycardia. SVT in utero can cause hydrops fetalis and intrauterine death and it is therefore treated in utero.

A 29. **A.** false **B.** false **C.** false **D.** false **E.** true

The Duckett-Jones major diagnostic criteria for rheumatic fever are carditis, polyarteritis, Syndenham's chorea, erythema marginatum and subcutaneous nodules.

A 30. **A.** true **B.** true **C.** true **D.** true **E.** true

The erythematous rash on the thenar and hypothenar eminence is known as Janeway lesions. Osler's nodes are painful hard embolic swellings on the extremities.

A 31. **A.** false **B.** true **C.** false **D.** false **E.** false

The classical features of nephrotic syndrome in the initial phases include periorbital oedema and lethargy. Diarrhoea may also be seen. Frothy urine is uncommon. The most common renal pathology is minimal change disease. Hyperlipidaemia is usually present, but is not part of the diagnostic triad of oedema, proteinuria and hypoalbuminaemia.

A 32. **A.** true **B.** false **C.** true **D.** true **E.** true

The four major features of acute nephritic syndrome are haematuria, proteinuria, oliguria and features of volume overload including oedema and hypertension.

A **33.** **A.** false   **B.** false   **C.** false   **D.** false   **E.** false

Complete heart block is present in about half of cases. It is associated with maternal anti-Rho antibodies, but most mothers are asymptomatic. The cutaneous features usually resolve after about 6 months.

A **34.** **A.** true   **B.** true   **C.** true   **D.** true   **E.** true

All of the listed infections may be associated with a vasculitis.

A **35.** **A.** true   **B.** false   **C.** false   **D.** false   **E.** false

Signs of valvular involvement are present within 2 weeks of illness in 80% of cases. The arthritis affects predominantly the large joints of the knees, ankles, elbows and wrists and responds very rapidly to salicylate therapy. Individual joints usually remain inflamed for less than a week only.

A **36.** **A.** false   **B.** false   **C.** true   **D.** false   **E.** false

Scheuermann's disease most commonly presents with mid-thoracic pain during the adolescent growth phase, though may be painless. It can also affect the thoracolumbar spine.

A **37.** **A.** false   **B.** false   **C.** true   **D.** false   **E.** false

In Perthes disease, the leg is semi-flexed and externally rotated at rest. It usually presents at age 4–10 years. It is bilateral in 10–20% of cases. Osteotomy is rarely required under age 6 years.

A **38.** **A.** false   **B.** false   **C.** false   **D.** true   **E.** true

Glue ear (or otitis media with effusion) requires fluid to persist in the middle ear for at least 8 weeks. Tympanometry shows a flat response as the tympanic membrane is non-mobile. Initial observation is generally done for 3 months prior to further intervention if necessary.

A **39.** **A.** false   **B.** false   **C.** true   **D.** false   **E.** false

Recurrent croup is most common in infants aged between 1 and 2 years. It responds to inhaled corticosteroids in the acute phase. *Staphylococcus aureus* causes pseudomembranous croup (bacterial tracheitis).

A 40. **A.** true **B.** false **C.** false **D.** false **E.** true

Bronchiolitis is usually due to the respiratory syncytial virus (RSV) but can be due to other viruses including parainfluenza viruses and rhinovirus. Apnoea occurs in about a fifth of infants admitted with bronchiolitis. Only one-third to a half of infants respond to bronchodilators. Recurrence is common.

A 41. **A.** true **B.** true **C.** false **D.** true **E.** false

Functional abdominal pain is usually paraumbilical and associated with good school performance in high-achieving girls. Pain that wakes the child at night or is associated with change in bowel habit or rectal mucus or bleeding, or with dysuria would suggest an organic cause.

A 42. **A.** true **B.** true **C.** false **D.** false **E.** false

Toddler food refusal is very common, and is a way for toddlers to exert their independence. It is helpful to remind parents of this, and that their child will not starve, to help them relax at mealtimes, which will in turn help the situation. It is best to introduce a wide variety of foods early during weaning, to have regular mealtimes, and not to insist that every meal is finished.

A 43. **A.** false **B.** true **C.** true **D.** true **E.** true

Boys are four times more likely than girls to have attention deficit hyperactivity disorder.

A 44. **A.** false **B.** true **C.** false **D.** false **E.** true

The antenatal nuchal scan is performed at 11–14 weeks. An increased nuchal fold thickness is indicative of Down's syndrome with a 77% sensitivity. There is a 5% false positive rate. Nuchal fold thickness when combined with maternal PAPP-A and inhibin levels has a 92% sensitivity rate, and this is further increased to 97% if the presence/absence of the nasal bone is added.

A 45. **A.** true **B.** true **C.** true **D.** false **E.** false

Intrauterine growth retardation and Down's syndrome are both causes of a decreased maternal serum alpha-fetoprotein level.

A **46.** **A.** false   **B.** false   **C.** false   **D.** false   **E.** false

Congenital dislocation of the hip should always be manually assessed in the examination of the newborn. In addition, if there are associated risk factors, a hip ultrasound and orthopaedic assessment are arranged. Due to the ductus arteriosus closing slowly during the first few days of life, cardiac disorders which are duct dependent may not present until duct closure. The Moro reflex is present from birth in a term baby. Meconium is passed by 24 hours of age in 95% of infants, and failure to do so is concerning of gut pathology. In some normal infants meconium may not be passed until 48 hours of age however.

A **47.** **A.** true   **B.** true   **C.** true   **D.** true   **E.** true

The Guthrie test is used to check universally for neonatal hypothyroidism and phenylketonuria. In addition it can be used to check for haemoglobinopathies, cystic fibrosis, HIV and certain rarer metabolic disorders.

A **48.** **A.** false   **B.** true   **C.** false   **D.** true   **E.** true

Facial nerve palsies are mostly lower motor neuron injuries secondary to forceps damage. The clavicle is the most common bone fractured, and is often undetected, healing on its own. Fractures of the humerus are usually of the upper third, and may cause a radial nerve injury.

A **49.** **A.** true   **B.** true   **C.** false   **D.** false   **E.** false

This is an infant with a conjugated hyperbilirubinaemia at 3 weeks of age. This may be due to neonatal hepatitis, biliary atresia, metabolic disease such as galactosaemia or sepsis. G6PD deficiency (with resulting haemolysis), bruising and breast milk jaundice result in an unconjugated hyperbilirubinaemia.

A **50.** **A.** true   **B.** true   **C.** false   **D.** false   **E.** true

Infants with neonatal hypothyroidism can be difficult to diagnose initially, and most are picked up on neonatal screening tests. The features however include hypotonia, a sleepy infant and feeding difficulties. Large fontanelles, a flat nasal bridge and widely spaced eyes may be present. Umbilical hernia, constipation, prolonged jaundice and abdominal distension are also features.

A 51. A. false **B.** false **C.** false **D.** true **E.** true

Diabetes insipidus may be central due to failure of release of antidiuretic hormone (ADH) caused by CNS disorders, or renal due to renal insensitivity to ADH (caused by intrinsic renal disease or various drugs). Cystic fibrosis, pneumonia and asthma can all cause SIADH.

A 52. A. true **B.** true **C.** true **D.** false **E.** true

Precocious puberty is a cause of tall stature during childhood because the growth spurts are reached earlier, but eventual adult height is short. Sotos syndrome ('cerebral gigantism') is a syndrome involving large hands, feet and ears, a prominent forehead and learning difficulties.

A 53. A. false **B.** true **C.** false **D.** false **E.** true

The first sign of puberty in boys is testicular enlargement. The timing and progress of puberty is very variable. Axillary hair appears before facial hair. The sebaceous glands are stimulated by adrenal androgens.

A 54. A. true **B.** false **C.** false **D.** true **E.** false

Tetracyclines can rarely cause the serious condition benign intracranial hypertension, features of which include headaches and visual disturbance. Tetracyclines are contraindicated in children under 12 years of age as they deposit in growing bones and teeth causing staining and sometimes dental hypoplasia. For this reason they should not be given to breast-feeding or pregnant women. Tetracyclines can exacerbate renal failure and so should not be given to children with kidney disease.

A 55. A. false **B.** false **C.** true **D.** false **E.** false

Metronidazole is present in large amounts in breast milk. Common side-effects are nausea and vomiting and other gastro-intestinal disturbances. Rarer side-effects are ataxia and a darkening of the urine. There is significant resistance with Giardiasis. The red man syndrome is caused by vancomycin.

A 56. A. false **B.** true **C.** false **D.** true **E.** false

Scarlet fever is due to a strain of Group A β-haemolytic Streptococcal infection which produces an erythrogenic exotoxin.

The entry site is usually the pharynx (after tonsillitis), and there is a sudden onset of fever, malaise and a 'white strawberry tongue' (white tongue with red papillae) followed by a 'strawberry tongue' (bright red tongue). It is treated with oral penicillin.

A 57. **A.** false **B.** false **C.** true **D.** false **E.** false

Rubella is infectious from a week before the onset of the rash. Initially there is a low-grade fever with conjunctivitis and cervical lymphadenopathy, and then a rash initially on the face, and then the whole body lasting a few days. Young children are often asymptomatic. The infection is most common during winter and spring.

A 58. **A.** false **B.** true **C.** false **D.** false **E.** false

Infectious mononucleosis has an incubation period of 20–30 days. It causes a fever, headache, tonsillitis, generalized lymphadenopathy, a rash, hepatitis, arthropathy and haematological abnormalities including haemolytic anaemia, thrombocytopenia and atypical lymphocytes. The splenomegaly is tender. The virus infects the B lymphocytes. In children under 5 years of age, the Monospot test (heterophile antigen to horse red blood cells) often gives false negative results.

A 59. **A.** false **B.** true **C.** false **D.** false **E.** true

Slapped cheek disease has a variable incubation period of between 4 and 21 days. It presents as a bright red rash on the cheeks and a lacy rash over the trunk and limbs which remits and recurs over up to several weeks. It is spread by droplet infection. An anaemia can occur in immunocompromised children.

A 60. **A.** true **B.** true **C.** false **D.** false **E.** false

Mumps infection may be spread via droplet or direct contact. It usually causes parotid swelling (mostly bilateral), and in a minority of cases submandibular swelling is seen. The incubation period is 14–21 days. It can cause trimus and hence interfere with eating.

A 61. **A.** false **B.** false **C.** false **D.** false **E.** false

None of these conditions are contraindications to childhood vaccination.

A **62.** **A.** false **B.** true **C.** false **D.** false **E.** false

Whole cell pertussis vaccine is an inactivated vaccine. It produces a better immunological response than acellular pertussis vaccine, and therefore was preferred for the primary course in children under 1 year. It should not be given to children over 1 year however because there is more likelihood of local side-effects than with the acellular pertussis vaccine. In a child with an evolving neurological condition, vaccination should be delayed until the prognosis is clear and specialist advice should be sought if there is any doubt.

A **63.** **A.** false **B.** true **C.** false **D.** false **E.** false

Diphtheria is a toxoid vaccine, and can be given to children who are immunosuppressed.

A **64.** **A.** false **B.** false **C.** false **D.** false **E.** false

A **65.** **A.** false **B.** false **C.** false **D.** true **E.** true

Varicella zoster (shingles) infection occurs from reactivation of dormant VZ virus. The rash is itchy and slightly painful in children. It is commonly seen in normal children. Aciclovir treatment is given if extensive or involving certain areas (e.g. the eye), or in immunocompromised children. Ramsay Hunt syndrome is infection of the geniculate ganglion causing ear pinna vesicles and facial nerve palsy.

Q 1. In a 10-year-old girl with headaches, which of the following clinical features would most concern you of underlying raised intracranial pressure

A. Visual field defects
B. Chronic rhinorrhoea
C. Worsening with chewing
D. Refractive errors
E. Hypertension

Q 2. The best advice to give a parent of a child with a neural tube defect is

A. Take low dose (5 mg) folic acid daily preconception
B. Take high dose folic acid (10 mg) daily preconception
C. Take high dose folic acid plus vitamin C daily preconception and during the first trimester
D. Take high dose folic acid preconception and during the first trimester
E. Take high dose folic acid preconception and during the pregnancy

Q 3. A meningomyelocele can cause

A. A neuropathic bladder
B. Neuropathic bowel
C. Scoliosis
D. Hydrocephalus
E. Hip dislocation

Q 4. Regarding neurofibromatosis type 1

A. Only 50% have a positive family history
B. It is autosomal recessive
C. Dental enamel pits are a feature
D. Café-au-lait macules are pathognomonic
E. Bilateral acoustic neuromas are a feature

Q 5. The following skills are normally acquired by the associated ages

A. Make circular scribbles – 18 months
B. Hop – 3.5 years
C. Stand on one leg – 3 years
D. Construct 2-word sentences – 2 years
E. Kick a ball – 2.5 years

Q 6. The age by which a normally developing child would have the ability to draw the following shapes are correctly matched

A. Circle – 2 years
B. Square – 3 years
C. Triangle – 4 years
D. Rhomboid – 5 years
E. Cross – 2 years

Q 7. The following abilities are correctly age-matched for a child who is developing normally

A. 3-cube tower – by 1 year
B. 8-cube tower – by 3 years
C. Climb upstairs on alternate feet – by 3 years
D. 6-cube tower – by 18 months
E. Bang cubes together – by 1 year

Q 8. A child with normal development should be able to do the following tasks by the associated ages

A. 3 to 4 word sentences – 2 years
B. Develops pincer grip – 6 months
C. Build a tower of 8 blocks – 4 years
D. Jump – 18 months
E. Builds a 3-cube bridge – 2 years

Q 9. A 5-year-old child developing normally can

A. Tie shoelaces
B. Do up buttons
C. Draw a diamond
D. Ride a bicycle
E. Say their surname

Q 10. **A normally developing 6-month-old infant offered a cube will be able to**

A. Throw it
B. Grasp it
C. Give it back
D. Reach for it
E. Transfer it from hand to hand

Q 11. **The following are features of Down's syndrome**

A. A tendency to mimicry
B. A good sense of rhythm
C. An increased incidence of Alzheimer's disease
D. Single transverse palmar crease in 80%
E. Brachydactyly in 75%

Q 12. **Features of normal newborns include**

A. A single transverse palmar crease in 10%
B. A bilateral transverse palmar crease in 1%
C. Umbilical hernia in 10% of black newborns
D. Epicanthic folds
E. Brushfield spots

Q 13. **The following are true**

A. Cystic fibrosis is the most common genetic lethal disease
B. A third sagittal fontanelle is present in 1 in 10 black infants
C. Low set ears are usually a normal feature in newborns
D. Pre-auricular tags are present in around 5% of newborns
E. Minor congenital malformations are present in 14% of newborns

Q 14. **Regarding cleft lip and palate**

A. The male:female ratio is 3:2
B. The incidence is 1 in 3000
C. The recurrence risk after one affected child is 1–2%
D. The recurrence risk after two affected children is 8–9%
E. The inheritance is autosomal dominant with variable penetrance

Q 15. Nasolacrimal duct obstruction

- **A.** Occurs in less than 1% of newborns
- **B.** Presents with a conjunctival injection
- **C.** Rarely resolves by 6 months
- **D.** Usually requires probing of the duct
- **E.** After 1 year of age may require silicone intubation

Q 16. Regarding leucocoria (white pupillary reflex)

- **A.** It may be caused by cataracts
- **B.** Retinoblastoma always produces it
- **C.** Marfan syndrome is associated
- **D.** It is associated with Down's syndrome
- **E.** It may be a normal finding in infancy

Q 17. Regarding accommodative convergent squint

- **A.** It occurs in association with myopia
- **B.** It is more noticeable when looking at close objects
- **C.** Corrective surgery is often required
- **D.** It usually develops during the first few months of life
- **E.** It can be brought on by bright sunlight

Q 18. In von Willebrand's disease

- **A.** It is transmitted by autosomal recessive inheritance
- **B.** The bleeding time is always normal
- **C.** Oral contraceptives can affect the symptoms
- **D.** The clinical features are very variable
- **E.** Menorrhagia is a feature

Q 19. Haemorrhagic disease of the newborn

- **A.** Is due to low levels of factor V
- **B.** Is of autosomal dominant inheritance
- **C.** Always develops during the first few days of life
- **D.** Is managed with prophylactic intramuscular or oral vitamin D
- **E.** Is associated with maternal diabetes mellitus

Q 20. Side-effects of minocycline therapy for acne include

- **A.** Depression
- **B.** Dry skin

C. Skin pigmentation

D. Hepatitis

E. Dental staining in children under 12 years

Q 21. Mongolian blue spots

A. Usually appears 2–3 weeks after birth

B. Are seen in about 10% of Asian babies

C. Are more common in Caucasian babies

D. Will fade completely during the first year of life

E. May be confused with non-accidental injury

Q 22. Impetigo

A. Is infection of the skin by *Staphylococcus aureus*

B. Rarely causes systemic upset in infants

C. Generally occurs as a complication of atopic eczema

D. May be bullous

E. Usually responds to topical antibiotics only

Q 23. Erythema multiforme

A. Is most commonly associated with inflammatory bowel disease

B. Generally requires treatment with topical steroids

C. May be recurrent

D. Is associated with dermatographism

E. May be caused by drugs

Q 24. Features of Marfan syndrome include

A. Hyperextensible joints

B. Downward lens dislocation

C. Striae

D. Mental retardation

E. Autosomal recessive inheritance

Q 25. The following are advantages of breast-feeding

A. Decreased incidence of osteoporosis

B. Decreased incidence of otitis media in the infant

C. Decreased incidence of ovarian cancer

D. More rapid maternal weight loss

E. Decreased incidence of uterine cancer

Q 26. Regarding rotavirus gastroenteritis

A. It has an incubation period of 5 days
B. A vaccine would not work
C. It presents with simultaneous onset of vomiting and diarrhoea
D. The gastrointestinal symptoms may be preceded by otitis media
E. The stools return to normal after 3 days

Q 27. The following are true of children with chronic constipation

A. Anal sphincter tone is increased
B. Diarrhoea is suggestive of an underlying aetiology such as coeliac disease
C. There is a male preponderance
D. Increased fat intake will increase gut velocity and aid in management
E. There is an association with cow's milk intolerance/allergy

Q 28. Common clinical signs of coarctation of the aorta in an older child are

A. Absent femoral pulses
B. Systolic murmur over the back
C. Systolic hypertension in the arms
D. Systolic murmur at the upper left sternal edge
E. Continuous murmur at the upper left sternal edge

Q 29. Maternal alcohol abuse is associated with fetal

A. Atrial septal defect
B. Ventricular septal defect
C. Patent ductus arteriosus
D. Ebstein anomaly
E. Coarctation of the aorta

Q 30. Tetralogy of Fallot is associated with

A. Down's syndrome
B. Maternal diabetes mellitus
C. DiGeorge syndrome

D. Williams syndrome

E. Lithium therapy

Q 31. The nephrotic syndrome

A. Presents with smoky-coloured urine

B. Causes polyuria

C. Is managed with antihypertensives

D. Always necessitates renal biopsy

E. Can be complicated by peritonitis

Q 32. In post-streptococcal glomerulonephritis

A. There is no proteinuria

B. Hypertension is a feature

C. Microscopic haematuria can persist

D. Penicillin treatment is necessary

E. C3 is low

Q 33. The following clinical features would indicate a possible diagnosis of systemic lupus erythematosis in a child with malaise, failure to thrive and arthralgia

A. A photosensitive rash

B. Heliotrope eyelid rash

C. Hypertension

D. Nailfold capillaritis

E. Subcutaneous calcium deposits

Q 34. The following are features of achondroplasia

A. Childhood obesity

B. Low IQ

C. Hypotonia in infancy

D. Otitis media

E. Hydrocephalus

Q 35. Causes of a positive antinuclear antibody (ANA) include

A. Juvenile idiopathic arthritis

B. Dermatomyositis

C. Normal population finding

D. SLE prior to any clinical features developing

E. Viral illness

Q 36. **The following are associated with in-toeing in toddlers**

    A. High arches
    B. Bow legs
    C. Knock knees
    D. Flat feet
    E. Metatarsus varus

Q 37. **Slipped upper femoral epiphysis (SUFE) is associated with**

    A. Tall, thin adolescent girls
    B. Fat boys
    C. Hyperthyroidism
    D. Hypogonadism
    E. Benign hypermobility syndrome

Q 38. **The following are indications for tonsillectomy**

    A. Recurrent tonsillitis with four or more episodes over 1 year
    B. Quinsy
    C. Obstructive sleep apnoea syndrome
    D. Episode of guttate psoriasis following tonsillitis
    E. Chronic otitis media

Q 39. **Bronchiolitis**

    A. Is most commonly seen in infants aged 6 months to 1 year old
    B. Is a cause of apnoea in small babies
    C. Usually lasts 1 week
    D. Is always caused by respiratory syncitial virus
    E. Is less common in rural areas

Q 40. **In pertussis infection**

    A. Most deaths are due to secondary bacterial pneumonia
    B. Erythromycin has no effect on the severity of the disease
    C. The initial catarrhal phase lasts 1–2 weeks
    D. Incubation is 3–7 days
    E. Infants do not always have the whoop

Q 41. **Which of the following features would make a seizure a more likely diagnosis than a breath-holding attack**

    A. Minor precipitating event
    B. Occurs in a child under 6 months of age

C. Cessation of breathing in expiration

D. Episode lasts more than 1 minute

E. Generalized seizure then cyanosis

Q 42. Regarding sleep disturbance in babies

A. Normal newborn infants sleep for 20 hours per day on average

B. Breast-fed infants sleep for shorter times than formula-fed infants

C. Breast-fed infants wake more frequently during the night than formula-fed infants

D. Sleepwalking occurs most commonly between ages 2 and 5 years

E. Infants sleep longer with fewer arousals when supine

Q 43. The following personality traits are associated with psychogenic eating disorders

A. Hyperactivity

B. High-achiever

C. Obsessional personality

D. High self-esteem

E. Learning disability

Q 44. The antenatal nuchal scan

A. Showing decreased nuchal fold thickness indicates an increased risk of Down's syndrome

B. May be combined with maternal PAPP-A and inhibin levels to increase accuracy

C. Is used to outline cervical integrity

D. Is 90% sensitive for Down's syndrome

E. Is an antenatal diagnostic test

Q 45. *Listeria monocytogenes* infection during pregnancy may cause

A. Hydrops fetalis

B. Premature delivery

C. Placental abruption

D. Neonatal seizures

E. Stillbirth

Q 46. **Neonatal umbilical cord infection**

  A. Is usually caused by *Haemophilus influenzae*
  B. Always requires intravenous antibiotic therapy
  C. Is often caused by *Klebsiella* infection
  D. Can cause bronchiectasis
  E. Can cause portal hypertension

Q 47. **Infants large for gestational age**

  A. Have a newborn weight above the 97th percentile
  B. Are more commonly born to mothers with pre-eclampsia
  C. Are at increased risk of hypoglycaemia
  D. Are at increased risk of polycythaemia
  E. Are at increased risk of hypothermia

Q 48. **Neonatal jaundice developing during the third week of life is likely to be due to**

  A. Congenital infection
  B. Hypothyroidism
  C. Severe bruising from birth
  D. Rhesus haemolytic disease
  E. Breast milk jaundice

Q 49. **Injury to the clavicle during delivery**

  A. Is the most common fracture due to delivery
  B. Is more common in infants of diabetic mothers
  C. Is more common in infants with neonatal lupus
  D. Should be treated by putting the infant's arm in a sling
  E. It is usually a greenstick fracture

Q 50. **Laboratory findings in the syndrome of inappropriate antidiuretic hormone secretion (SIADH) are**

  A. Hyponatraemia with elevated plasma osmolality
  B. Plasma osmolality elevated compared to urine osmolality
  C. Low urine sodium concentration for the serum hyponatraemia
  D. Hypochloraemia
  E. Hyperkalaemia

Q 51. Regarding polycystic ovary syndrome

A. The ovaries are of normal size
B. There is insulin resistance
C. Obesity is a cardinal feature
D. There is a low LH:FSH ratio
E. Acne is a feature

Q 52. Normal puberty findings include

A. Earlier onset in girls on average
B. Adrenarche the first sign of onset in boys
C. Menarche the first sign of onset in girls
D. Testicular volume of 6 ml is prepubertal
E. Onset of menstruation at an average age of 11.5 years

Q 53. Precocious puberty

A. May be caused by anorexia nervosa
B. Is seen in Turner syndrome
C. May be caused by a prolactin-secreting tumour
D. Is twice as common in girls
E. May be caused by radiotherapy for ALL

Q 54. Trimethoprim

A. May be used with caution during breast-feeding
B. May cause blood dyscrasias with long-term therapy
C. Commonly causes nausea
D. Is used in the treatment of Giardiasis
E. Is an aminoglycoside

Q 55. Sodium valproate

A. Is effective in the treatment of absence seizures
B. Causes gum hypertrophy
C. Can cause liver toxicity
D. Is associated with neonatal bleeding
E. Is associated with neural tube defects if taken during pregnancy

Q 56. Regarding lymphadenitis in an otherwise healthy child

A. It is most commonly due to Group A haemolytic Streptococcal infection

B. It may be due to *Bartonella henselae*

C. Swollen non-tender lymphadenitis is suggestive of cat scratch disease

D. A red non-tender indurated submandibular node is suggestive of mycobacterium infection

E. It is rarely due to *Staphylococcus aureus* infection

Q 57. In otitis media

A. The most common bacterial cause is *Streptococcus pneumoniae*

B. Ear pulling is a reliable clinical sign of otitis media in toddlers

C. It rarely resolves spontaneously

D. 25% of children will have a middle ear effusion 2 weeks after the acute infection

E. 10% of children have a middle ear effusion 1 month after the acute infection

Q 58. Regarding fever in infancy

A. Axillary temperature is 1.5 °C lower than rectal temperature

B. Tympanic temperature is the same as rectal temperature

C. Otitis media increases the reading of tympanic temperature significantly

D. Teething causes temperature elevation

E. Tympanic temperature readings are reliable in infants under 3 months old

Q 59. Roseola infantum

A. Is caused by Parvovirus B19

B. Presents with a prodromal low-grade fever and pharyngitis

C. May cause seizures in the eruptive phase

D. Is a common cause of febrile convulsions

E. Often has associated diarrhoea

Q 60. Cat scratch fever

A. Is caused by a virus

B. Has a 1-week incubation period

C. Is transmitted primarily from kittens

D. Causes a generalized maculopapular rash

E. Resolves spontaneously

Q 61. **The following are contraindications to childhood vaccination**

   A. Stable neurological condition

   B. Chronic disease

   C. Previous mumps infection

   D. Treatment with topical steroids

   E. Severe atopic eczema

Q 62. **Tetanus vaccination**

   A. Is a live vaccine

   B. Should not be given to a child who had a severe local reaction to the previous tetanus vaccination

   C. May be given to a child on high dose steroid therapy

   D. Cannot be given to a child receiving radiotherapy

   E. Cannot be given to a child with leukaemia

Q 63. **The following are killed organism vaccines**

   A. Typhoid

   B. Influenza

   C. The BCG

   D. Yellow fever

   E. Rabies

Q 64. **Live vaccines**

   A. Can be given to children on high dose oral steroids

   B. Can be given to children who received chemotherapy after an interval of 3 months

   C. Can be given to children with hypogammaglobulinaemia

   D. Can be given within 2 weeks of another live vaccine

   E. Should not be given within 3 months of receiving immunoglobulin

Q 65. **The following are common causes of wheeze in childhood**

   A. Bronchiolitis

   B. Cystic fibrosis

   C. Whooping cough

   D. Heart failure

   E. Viral induced wheeze

A 1. **A.** true **B.** false **C.** false **D.** false **E.** false

A 2. **A.** false **B.** false **C.** false **D.** true **E.** false

A 3. **A.** true **B.** true **C.** true **D.** true **E.** true

Hip dislocation occurs secondary to muscular imbalance.

A 4. **A.** true **B.** false **C.** false **D.** false **E.** false

Neurofibromatosis is autosomal dominant, however due to the high spontaneous mutation rate only half have a positive family history. Dental enamel pits are a features of tuberous sclerosis. Café-au-lait macules are a feature of several conditions including neurofibromatosis type 1. Bilateral acoustic neuromas are a feature of neurofibromatosis type 2.

A 5. **A.** false **B.** false **C.** false **D.** true **E.** false

A normal child can make circular scribbles and kick a ball by 2 years, and stand on one leg and hop by 4 years.

A 6. **A.** false **B.** false **C.** false **D.** false **E.** false

The age by which most children can draw the shapes are as follows: a circle by 3 years, a square by 4.5 years, a triangle by 5 years, a rhomboid by 7 years and a cross by 4 years.

A 7. **A.** false **B.** true **C.** true **D.** false **E.** false

A normally developing child can build a 3-cube tower by 18 months, a 6-cube tower by 2 years and an 8-cube tower by 3 years.

A 8. **A.** false **B.** false **C.** false **D.** false **E.** false

Children developing normally should be able to build a tower of 8 blocks, have 3–4 word sentences and jump by 3 years. A normal child has pincer grip by 9 months and can build a 3-cube bridge by 3 years.

A 9. **A.** true **B.** true **C.** false **D.** true **E.** true

The ability to draw a diamond develops by age 7 years.

A 10. **A.** false **B.** true **C.** false **D.** true **E.** true

A 6-month-old infant may drop the cube, but not throw it. An infant will give objects back from around 1 year of age.

A 11. **A.** true **B.** true **C.** true **D.** false **E.** false

Only around 50% of Down's syndrome patients have a single transverse palmar crease and the same proportion have brachydactyly.

A 12. **A.** false **B.** true **C.** false **D.** true **E.** true

A single transverse palmar crease is present in around 4% of newborns. Umbilical hernias are present in 6% of newborn black infants. Brushfield spots are seen in normal infants, most commonly in Caucasians.

A 13. **A.** true **B.** true **C.** true **D.** false **E.** true

Pre-auricular tags are rare, occurring in less than 1% of newborns.

A 14. **A.** true **B.** false **C.** false **D.** true **E.** true

The incidence is 1 in 1000. The recurrence risk after one affected child is 3–4%. The inheritance is polygenic.

A 15. **A.** false **B.** false **C.** false **D.** false **E.** true

Nasolacrimal duct obstruction is a relatively frequent condition in infants, occurring in around 5% of babies. It presents with a watering eye and a clear conjunctiva. Gentle massage of the area is helpful. Usually the obstruction resolves spontaneously by 6 months of age. Infants over 1 year should be seen by an ophthalmologist and probing of the duct is usually successful. Over 1 year of age, silicone intubation may be necessary.

A **16.** **A.** true   **B.** false   **C.** false   **D.** true   **E.** false

Leucocoria is always pathological. It may be caused by cataracts, and hence is associated with Down's syndrome (as is cataract). In only around 70% of cases does retinoblastoma present with leucocoria.

A **17.** **A.** false   **B.** true   **C.** false   **D.** false   **E.** false

Accommodative convergent squint usually develops between age 2 and 4 years. It occurs in hyperopic (long-sighted) children as they try to focus on a close object and there is an imbalance between accommodation and convergence. It usually resolves with glasses to correct the refractive error.

A **18.** **A.** false   **B.** false   **C.** true   **D.** true   **E.** true

Von Willebrand's disease is actually a group of disorders involving the von Willebrand factor (vWF). The clinical features within and between the different types vary. The inheritance is autosomal dominant. The bleeding time is prolonged, but may be normal in mild disease.

A **19.** **A.** false   **B.** false   **C.** false   **D.** false   **E.** false

Haemorrhagic disease of the newborn is a rare but potentially catastrophic disorder due to low vitamin K-dependent clotting factors (i.e. factors II, VII, IX and X). Prophylactic vitamin K is given to all neonates with parental approval, either as a single intramuscular injection or as three oral doses. It usually presents in the first week of life but can rarely present late at around 6 weeks.

A **20.** **A.** false   **B.** false   **C.** true   **D.** true   **E.** true

Skin pigmentation may be irreversible. Minocycline is contraindicated in children under 12 years of age due to the dental effects, which are permanent.

A **21.** **A.** false   **B.** false   **C.** false   **D.** false   **E.** true

Mongolian blue spot(s) are present at birth and gradually become less apparent over many years. They are much more frequently seen in Asian and black babies (present in about 80% of Asian babies) than Caucasian babies. They can appear like bruising and be confused with non-accidental injury.

A **22.** **A.** false **B.** false **C.** false **D.** true **E.** false

Impetigo is due to skin infection with staphylococci or streptococci, or both. It classically causes honey-coloured crusts to develop, but a bullous form due to a particular *Staphylococcus* is seen. It occurs in children with normal skin, but may complicate atopic eczema. It is very contagious. The child is usually well, but infants in particular may be unwell. It is usually treated with oral antibiotics.

A **23.** **A.** false **B.** false **C.** true **D.** false **E.** true

Erythema multiforme is a rash typically of target lesions, and most commonly due to herpes simplex infection, though it may be post-infectious or drug-induced (particularly by sulphonamides). It usually resolves spontaneously.

A **24.** **A.** true **B.** false **C.** true **D.** false **E.** false

Marfan syndrome is an autosomal dominant condition with abnormal fibrillin in the connective tissue. The features include tall stature and arachnodactyly. Cardiac defects include mitral valve prolapse, aortic regurgitation and aneurysms. There is a risk of sudden death from ruptured aortic aneurysm. Lens dislocation is classically upwards. Intelligence is normal.

A **25.** **A.** true **B.** true **C.** true **D.** true **E.** false

Breast-feeding gives a protection from breast cancer of 4.7% per year breast-feeding, and also protects against ovarian cancer. There is more rapid uterine involution and increased post-partum weight loss.

A **26.** **A.** false **B.** false **C.** false **D.** true **E.** false

Rotavirus is the most common cause of gastroenteritis in children. The incubation period is 24–48 hours. In about half of cases there is an initial respiratory illness including otitis media. Vomiting for 1–3 days is followed by diarrhoea, which may last for about a week.

A 27. **A.** false **B.** false **C.** false **D.** false **E.** false

Anal sphincter tone is increased in Hirschsprung's disease. Overflow diarrhoea can occur with simple chronic constipation and does not indicate necessarily any other underlying pathology. Fat will slow GI transit time and increased fluid and fibre should be recommended.

Murphey S, Claydon G. Chapter 20. In *Pediatric Gastrointestinal Disease.* Ed. Walker A *et al.* St Louis: Mosby, 1996.

A 28. **A.** false **B.** true **C.** true **D.** false **E.** false

The femoral pulses are usually weak, but very rarely absent.

A 29. **A.** true **B.** true **C.** false **D.** false **E.** true

Features of fetal alcohol syndrome are dysmorphism (long philtrum, flat nasal bridge, midfacial hypoplasia, micrognathia, upturned nose, ear deformities, eye malformations and cleft lip and palate), microcephaly and developmental delay, growth retardation, and renal and limb abnormalities. The cardiac defects associated are VSD, ASD and coarctation of the aorta.

A 30. **A.** true **B.** false **C.** true **D.** false **E.** false

Tetralogy of Fallot is associated with Down's syndrome and DiGeorge syndrome.

A 31. **A.** false **B.** false **C.** false **D.** false **E.** true

The nephrotic syndrome is characterized by proteinuria with hypoalbuminaemia and oedema. The urine may be frothy if there is large protein loss, and there may be oliguria due to the intravascular hypovolaemia that occurs. Management is initially with oral steroids. Renal biopsy is only indicated in cases which fail to respond to steroids or with atypical features.

A 32. **A.** false **B.** true **C.** true **D.** true **E.** false

Post-streptococcal glomerulonephritis occurs 2–3 weeks after streptococcal infection; usually a throat or skin infection. The features are haematuria, proteinuria, oliguria and volume overload leading to hypertension. Microscopic haematuria can continue for up to 1 year. C3 is raised and C4 is normal.

A **33.** **A.** true **B.** false **C.** true **D.** false **E.** false

A heliotrope eyelid rash, nailfold capillaritis and subcutaneous calcium deposits are classically seen in juvenile dermatomyositis.

A **34.** **A.** true **B.** false **C.** true **D.** true **E.** true

Achondroplasia is the most common skeletal dysplasia. The features are short stature, megalocephaly, low nasal bridge, prominent forehead, midfacial hypoplasia and narrow nasal passages, lumbar lordosis, short humeri, trident hands. There is mild hypotonia in infancy, and increased incidence of hydrocephalus (secondary to a narrow foramen magnum), otitis media, and childhood obesity. Intelligence is normal.

A **35.** **A.** true **B.** true **C.** true **D.** true **E.** true

A positive ANA is found in response to viral infections and as part of the normal population in addition to rheumatological disorders. It is important therefore to check the titre, and to repeat the test at a later date if necessary.

A **36.** **A.** false **B.** true **C.** true **D.** true **E.** true

Metatarsus varus may need surgery. It is also associated with internal tibial torsion, metatarsus adductus and spasticity.

A **37.** **A.** true **B.** true **C.** false **D.** true **E.** false

Slipped upper femoral epiphysis (SUFE) is seen in both fat boys with relative hypogonadism and tall, thin girls with increased growth hormone. It is associated with hypogonadism, hypothyroidism and pituitary dysfunction.

A **38.** **A.** false **B.** false **C.** true **D.** false **E.** false

The current widely agreed indications for tonsillectomy are at least six attacks per year for 2 years or at least three attacks per year over a number of years for the older child, and obstructive sleep apnoea syndrome.

A **39.** **A.** false **B.** true **C.** false **D.** false **E.** true

Bronchiolitis is usually due to infection with respiratory syncytial virus (RSV) but can be due to other viruses. It is most common in infants under 6 months of age, and generally lasts about 3 weeks.

A **40.** **A.** true **B.** false **C.** true **D.** false **E.** true

About 90% of the deaths are due to pneumonia, most of which is secondary bacterial infection that can easily be missed during the paroxysmal phase as the respiratory symptoms are so prominent then. Erythromycin reduces the severity of paroxysmal symptoms if given within 2 weeks of illness, but should be given at any stage as it prevents spread to others. The incubation period is 7–14 days.

A **41.** **A.** true **B.** true **C.** false **D.** true **E.** true

Breath-holding attacks are characterized by intense crying, stopping breathing in expiration, then pallor, then cyanosis and rigidity and then loss of consciousness and a generalized tonic-clonic seizure may occur. The seizure is preceded by the cyanosis.

A **42.** **A.** false **B.** true **C.** true **D.** false **E.** false

Normal newborn infants sleep for 16 hours per day on average. Sleepwalking occurs most commonly between ages 5 and 10 years. Infants sleep longer with fewer arousals when prone.

A **43.** **A.** false **B.** true **C.** true **D.** false **E.** false

The typical personality profile of a child with a psychogenic eating disorder include a high-achiever, poor self-esteem, depression and obsessional traits (in particular thoughts of body shape and food).

A **44.** **A.** false **B.** true **C.** true **D.** false **E.** false

The antenatal nuchal scan is a screening procedure. Assessment of nuchal fold thickness gives an estimated risk of Down's syndrome, not an actual diagnosis. An increased nuchal fold thickness is associated with Down's syndrome. The sensitivity of the scan is 77%, but this is increased to 92% with addition of maternal PAPP-A and inhibin levels. Assessment of the uteroplacental circulation, cervical integrity and early anomaly scan and diagnosis of twins is also possible at this scan.

A **45.** **A.** false **B.** true **C.** false **D.** true **E.** true

Listeria monocytogenes infection during pregnancy can be catastrophic. It is acquired from unpasteurized products, soft cheeses, chicken, raw vegetables, uncooked meats and reheated foods. Premature delivery, abortion or stillbirth may occur. Neonatal infection causing pneumonia or disseminated infection causing fits and later hydrocephalus may occur.

A **46.** **A.** false **B.** false **C.** true **D.** false **E.** true

The predominant organisms are *Staphylococcus aureus* and *Escherichia coli*, and in addition *Klebsiella* and *Pseudomonas* may cause it. Intravenous antibiotics may be necessary if there are signs of spread (i.e. cellulitis). The infection can spread via the haematogenous route and cause portal vein phlebitis with later development of portal hypertension.

A **47.** **A.** false **B.** false **C.** true **D.** true **E.** false

Infants who are large for gestational age are defined as those over the 90th percentile for weight. They are at increased risk of birth trauma, hypoglycaemia and polycythaemia. Maternal pre-eclampsia is associated with intrauterine growth retardation.

A **48.** **A.** false **B.** false **C.** false **D.** false **E.** true

Rhesus haemolytic disease and congenital infection will cause jaundice during the first 24 hours usually. Severe bruising from birth and hypothyroidism will usually cause jaundice to develop before the third week.

A **49.** **A.** true **B.** true **C.** false **D.** false **E.** true

Fracture of the clavicle is due to excessive traction during the delivery. It is usually a greenstick fracture, and is the most common fracture during delivery. It is more common in large infants (e.g. those born to mothers with diabetes).

A **50.** **A.** false **B.** false **C.** false **D.** true **E.** false

In the syndrome of inappropriate antidiuretic hormone secretion (SIADH) the plasma osmolality, sodium and chloride are low. The urine sodium is inappropriately high and urine osmolality is normal.

A **51.** **A.** false **B.** true **C.** false **D.** false **E.** true

In polycystic ovary syndrome the ovaries are large with multiple peripheral cysts. The features include irregular menses or secondary amenorrhoea, hirsutism, acne and insulin resistance. While obesity may be present, in many cases weight is within normal limits. Circulating androgen levels and the LH:FSH ratio high.

A 52. **A.** true **B.** false **C.** false **D.** false **E.** false

The first sign of puberty in boys is testicular enlargement, and in girls is breast development. A testicular volume of 4 ml indicates onset of puberty. The average age of menstruation onset is 12.2 years.

A 53. **A.** true **B.** false **C.** false **D.** false **E.** true

Precocious puberty is approximately 5–10 times more common in girls than boys. Prolactin-secreting tumours and Turner syndrome are both causes of delayed puberty. Cranial radiotherapy used in ALL may result in precocious puberty.

A 54. **A.** true **B.** true **C.** true **D.** false **E.** false

The short-term use of trimethoprim during breast-feeding is not known to be harmful. It is present in small amounts in breast milk. Depression of haematopoiesis can occur and parents of children on long-term therapy should be advised to recognize the signs of blood disorders.

A 55. **A.** true **B.** false **C.** true **D.** false **E.** true

Sodium valproate is used in the treatment of generalized tonic-clonic seizures and absence seizures. Phenytoin causes gum hypertrophy. One of the main side-effects of sodium valproate is liver toxicity, and is particularly seen in children under 3 years of age. Carbamazepine and phenytoin are associated with neonatal bleeding.

A 56. **A.** false **B.** true **C.** false **D.** true **E.** false

Lymphadenitis in an otherwise healthy child is most commonly due to *Staphylococcus aureus*. *Bartonella henselae* causes cat scratch disease, which is characterized by tender lymphadenopathy.

A 57. **A.** true **B.** false **C.** false **D.** false **E.** false

Ear pulling is not a reliable indicator of otitis media in the absence of other symptoms and signs. 70% of children have a middle ear effusion 2 weeks after the acute infection, and 20% will still have an effusion 2 months after the acute infection. In over 50% of cases, otitis media will resolve spontaneously.

A **58.** **A.** false   **B.** false   **C.** false   **D.** true   **E.** false

The axillary temperature is 0.8–1.0 °C lower than rectal temperature, and tympanic temperature is 0.5–0.6 °C lower. Otitis media can increase tympanic temperature recordings very slightly (by only about 0.1 °C). Teething can cause a modest temperature rise (to 37.5 °C). Children under 3 months old have narrow ear canals which can collapse, resulting in tympanic temperature readings recording the cooler canal temperature and not the tympanic temperature.

A **59.** **A.** false   **B.** false   **C.** false   **D.** true   **E.** true

Roseola infantum is caused by HHV-6. It presents with a sudden onset high fever, during which time seizures may be seen (the pre-eruptive phase). It is thought to be the cause of up to one-third of febrile convulsions in children under 2 years of age.

A **60.** **A.** false   **B.** false   **C.** true   **D.** false   **E.** true

Cat scratch fever is caused by the Gram-negative bacillus *Bartonella henselae*. It is spread by a scratch or contact from cats but especially kittens. The incubation period is from 3 to 30 days. The cardinal clinical features are an inoculation papule or pustule (not present in up to half of cases), and regional lymphadenopathy which lasts up to 2–4 months. It often resolves spontaneously, but antibiotics are effective in severe disease.

A **61.** **A.** false   **B.** false   **C.** false   **D.** false   **E.** false

None of the conditions are contraindications to childhood vaccination.

A **62.** **A.** false   **B.** false   **C.** true   **D.** false   **E.** false

Tetanus is not a live vaccine, and therefore can be given to immunosuppressed children, including those with malignancy and those on immunosuppressive therapy. A severe local reaction to a previous dose is not a contraindication to further doses.

A **63.** **A.** true   **B.** true   **C.** false   **D.** false   **E.** true

Yellow fever and the BCG are both live vaccines.

A **64.** **A.** false   **B.** false   **C.** false   **D.** false   **E.** true

Live vaccines cannot be given to children on high dose steroids, to children with impaired immunity (e.g. hypogammaglobulinaemia) or within 3 weeks of another live vaccine (unless given simultaneously). They should not be given to children receiving chemotherapy until at least 6 months after treatment has ceased.

A **65.** **A.** true   **B.** false   **C.** false   **D.** false   **E.** true

Since the immunization against pertussis was introduced, this is an uncommon condition.

Exam 5

Answers

'Best of five' questions

FOR EACH QUESTION, SELECT ONE ANSWER ONLY

Q 1. A 10-year-old girl has been having episodes of abdominal pain causing her to be off school every few weeks for the last few months. The pain is periumbilical. She is of normal weight and otherwise well. What is the most probable diagnosis?

    A. Anorexia nervosa
    B. Constipation
    C. Migraine
    D. Non-organic abdominal pain
    E. Chronic appendicitis

Q 2. A 5-year-old boy was found to have multiple café-au-lait macules and axillary freckling on examination. Which of the following is the most important investigation to do?

    A. Full blood count
    B. MRI brain scan
    C. Skin biopsy
    D. Chest X-ray
    E. Electroencephalogram

Extended matching questions

Q 1. The following is a list of diagnoses

    A. Roseola infantum
    B. Parvovirus B19
    C. Hand, foot and mouth disease
    D. Cat scratch disease

E. Measles

F. Chicken pox

Choose the most likely diagnosis in the following case

A 2-year-old infant had developed a sudden fever of 39.5 °C with mild coryza but was otherwise well. The fever settled and 3 days later a macular erythema developed over the trunk and arms. Examination was otherwise unremarkable except for slight cervical lymphadenopathy.

Q 2. **The following is a list of diagnoses**

A. Childhood absence epilepsy

B. Infantile spasms

C. Temporal lobe epilepsy

D. Benign intracranial hypertension

E. Benign paroxysmal vertigo

F. Breath-holding attacks

Choose the most likely diagnosis in the following case

A 14-year-old girl on the oral contraceptive pill complains of double vision. Marked papilloedema is noted on examination.

'Best of five' questions

A 1. D.

Recurrent abdominal pain is due to non-organic reasons in about 90% of cases, but should be investigated as it is necessary to exclude organic causes.

A 2. B.

This boy has features of neurofibromatosis. The pertinent investigations include blood pressure, height and weight check, and a brain scan to exclude intracranial lesions.

Extended matching questions

A 1. A.

Roseola infantum is caused by human-herpes virus 6. The clinical features are a high fever and mild coryza, cervical lymphadenopathy with later a red macular rash over the face, trunk and arms. Febrile convulsions may occur. Only around a one-third of cases are symptomatic however.

A 2. D.

Benign intracranial hypertension presents with features of chronic raised intracranial pressure. Infarction of the optic nerve may occur with subsequent blindness if not swiftly treated. The known causes include the oral contraceptive pill, isotretinoin, tertracyclines and steroid withdrawal.

'Best of five' questions

FOR EACH QUESTION, SELECT ONE ANSWER ONLY

Q 1. A 2-month-old infant has developed two chest infections since birth. His mother complains he has bad possetting and is irritable in the evenings particularly. What is the most probable diagnosis?

   A. Cystic fibrosis
   B. Gastoenteritis
   C. Congenital diaphragmatic hernia
   D. Gastro-oesophageal reflux
   E. Congenital immunodeficiency

Q 2. A 9-month-old baby presents to casualty with an 8-hour history of lethargy and has a purpuric rash. What is the best immediate management option?

   A. Do a lumbar puncture
   B. Give intravenous broad-spectrum antibiotics
   C. Do a CT brain scan
   D. Send to intensive care unit
   E. Insert an interosseous needle

Extended matching questions

Q 1. The following is a list of diagnoses

   A. Roseola infantum
   B. Parvovirus B19
   C. Hand, foot and mouth disease
   D. Cat scratch disease
   E. Measles
   F. Chicken pox

Choose the most likely diagnosis for the following case

A 5-year-old boy had a coryza and headache and a fever of 38.2 °C. On examination, he had erythematous cheeks and a lacy erythematous rash on the trunk and upper limbs.

Q 2. The following is a list of diagnoses

A. Childhood absence epilepsy

B. Infantile spasms

C. Temporal lobe epilepsy

D. Benign intracranial hypertension

E. Benign paroxysmal vertigo

F. Breath-holding attacks

Choose the most likely diagnosis in the following case

A toddler, whilst having his tea, becomes very cross when asked to eat his yoghurt and becomes pale and then stiffens with clonic movements, then goes slightly limp and quickly recovers.

'Best of five' questions

A 1.   **D.**

Gastro-oesophageal reflux can present with possetting and distress particularly noticeable in the evening. If severe, inhalation results in chest infections developing.

A 2.   **B.**

This infant has features of meningococcal sepsis. The immediate management is to resuscitate as necessary, via intravenous (or if necessary interosseous) access and to give broad-spectrum intravenous antibiotics to cover the most likely pathogen as the mortality is related to the exponential growth of the bacteria and the sooner the infection is treated the better.

Extended matching questions

A 1.   **B.**

Parvovirus B19 causes slapped cheek disease, which is most commonly seen in school age children during the spring. Children with chronic haemolysis including those with sickle cell anaemia and thalassaemia major can get a transient aplastic crisis as the virus attacks the red cell precursors leading to a transient arrest of erythropoiesis.

A 2.   **F.**

Breath-holding attacks are seen in toddlers precipitated by emotion (anger or fear). The child cries then becomes blue or pale, then stiffens with clonic movements, then goes slightly limp and quickly recovers.

'Best of five' questions

FOR EACH QUESTION, SELECT <u>ONE</u> ANSWER ONLY

Q 1. A 6-week-old boy develops severe projectile vomiting. He has been losing weight and is constantly hungry. What is the most probable diagnosis?

A. Severe gastro-oesophageal reflux
B. Pyloric stenosis
C. Crohn's disease
D. Hirschsprung's disease
E. Constipation

Q 2. A 3-week-old breast-fed infant presents with jaundice and is feeding well. What is the most likely cause of the jaundice?

A. Bruising
B. Hypothyroidism
C. Urinary tract infection
D. Rhesus incompatibility
E. Breast milk jaundice

Extended matching questions

Q 1. The following is a list of diagnoses

A. Roseola infantum
B. Parvovirus B19
C. Hand, foot and mouth disease
D. Cat scratch disease
E. Measles
F. Chicken pox

Choose the most likely diagnosis in the following case

A 2-year-old infant developed a low-grade fever and a generalized maculopapular rash and vesicles on the tongue, buccal mucosa and palms.

Q 2.   The following is a list of diagnoses

A. Childhood absence epilepsy
B. Infantile spasms
C. Temporal lobe epilepsy
D. Benign intracranial hypertension
E. Benign paroxysmal vertigo
F. Breath-holding attacks

Choose the most likely diagnosis in the following case

A 4-month-old infant develops frequent short bursts of sudden symmetrical contractions accompanied by apparent loss of awareness. There is concern regarding the infant's development.

'Best of five' questions

A 1. B.

Pyloric stenosis is due to hypertrophy of the pylorus and presents between 2 and 7 weeks of age, most commonly in boys. The features are projectile vomiting, consequent hunger and weight loss. The infants have a hypochloraemic alkalosis.

A 2. E.

Breast milk jaundice or physiological jaundice are the most common cause of jaundice in a healthy (breast-fed) infant after 2 weeks of age. This jaundice is due to unconjugated bilirubin, and this needs to be confirmed.

Extended matching questions

A 1. C.

Hand, foot and mouth disease is due to enteroviral infection including Coxsackie A or B. It may be spread via faecal-oral or droplet route, or by direct contact. The disease is usually seen in pre-school children. It causes a mild illness with fever, vesicles in the mouth, palms and to a lesser extent the soles, and a generalized maculopapular rash, particularly with papules on the buttocks.

A 2. B.

Infantile spasms are generalized seizures developing usually from 4 to 6 months of age. They are associated with arrested development and need thorough investigation to search for a cause.

'Best of five' questions

FOR EACH QUESTION, SELECT <u>ONE</u> ANSWER ONLY

Q 1. **A 2-year-old child has smelly stools and abdominal distension. His growth has been poor since around 10 months of age. What is the most probable diagnosis?**

A. Coeliac disease
B. Crohn's disease
C. Irritable bowel syndrome
D. Giardiasis
E. Abdominal migraine

Q 2. **A 6-month-old boy has bilateral undescended testes. The best initial course of action is to**

A. Review in 3 months time
B. Give human chorionic gonadotrophin (HCG) injections
C. Do an orchidopexy
D. Do an ultrasound scan of the pelvis and inguinal canal
E. Do an orchidectomy

Extended matching questions

Q 1. **The following is a list of diagnoses**

A. Roseola infantum
B. Parvovirus B19
C. Hand, foot and mouth disease
D. Cat scratch disease
E. Measles
F. Chicken pox

Choose the most likely diagnosis in the following case

An 11-month-old infant had a 2-day history of cough, coryza and conjunctivitis. He was lethargic and had a fever of 39.9 °C and a generalized fine red maculopapular rash.

Q 2. **The following is a list of diagnoses**

A. Childhood absence epilepsy

B. Infantile spasms

C. Temporal lobe epilepsy

D. Benign intracranial hypertension

E. Benign paroxysmal vertigo

F. Breath-holding attacks

Choose the most likely diagnosis in the following case

A 5-year-old boy is noticed to have episodes of inattention accompanied by eyelid fluttering lasting approximately 1 minute. These are frequently associated with hunger or stress.

Supplementary Answers

'Best of five' questions

A 1. A.

Coeliac disease may manifest when the child is weaned, and thus begins eating gluten, usually from about 6 months of age, although often presents much later, even in adult life. The classical symptoms of the smelly stools and abdominal distension are not always present. The consequent malabsorption results in a slow down in growth.

A 2. D.

The initial course of action is to do an USS to see if the testes are located in the inguinal canal. If they are not, a laparoscopy may be necessary to identify if they are intra-abdominal, or indeed present at all.

Extended matching questions

A 1. E.

Measles is spread by droplet infection. The incubation period is 7–14 days. Initially there are coryzal symptoms with cough and conjunctivitis and a high fever. The rash appears around day 2–3 of the illness. The classical Koplik's spots may be seen opposite the second molar.

A 2. A.

Childhood absence epilepsy is most common from 3 to 10 years of age, and there is a family history in 40% of cases. The seizure usually lasts around 30 seconds when there is a sudden loss of awareness with no motor activity, which may be accompanied by eyelid fluttering. Seizures may be induced by emotion, hunger or hyperventilation.

'Best of five' questions

FOR EACH QUESTION, SELECT ONE ANSWER ONLY

Q 1. A 15-month-old girl develops bilateral breast enlargement. She had no axillary or pubic hair. Her height was in the mid-parental range. What is the most probable diagnosis?

    A. Klinefelter's syndrome
    B. Precocious puberty
    C. Premature thelarche
    D. Congenital adrenal hyperplasia
    E. Hyperthyroidism

Q 2. A 2-day-old newborn infant has a generalized rash of red papules, some with a white pinpoint pustular centre. The baby is breast-feeding well and there are no other symptoms. What is the most likely diagnosis?

    A. Acropustulosis
    B. Staphylococcal sepsis
    C. Erythema toxicum neonatorum
    D. Congenital herpes simplex infection
    E. Congenital varicella

Extended matching questions

Q 1. The following is a list of diagnoses

    A. Roseola infantum
    B. Parvovirus B19
    C. Hand, foot and mouth disease
    D. Cat scratch disease

E. Measles

F. Chicken pox

Choose the most likely diagnosis in the following cases

A. A 6-year-old girl developed mild malaise and a fever of 38.1 °C but was otherwise well. On examination she had extensive left axillary lymphadenopathy. She had a history of a pustule on the left forearm 1 week previously.

B. An 18-month-old infant had a 48-hour history of fever and malaise, followed by an itchy papular rash in the post-auricular area, which had spread to the head, face and upper trunk. Some of the lesions had become vesicular.

Q 2. **The following is a list of diagnoses**

A. Childhood absence epilepsy

B. Infantile spasms

C. Temporal lobe epilepsy

D. Benign intracranial hypertension

E. Benign paroxysmal vertigo

F. Breath-holding attacks

Choose the most likely diagnosis in the following case

A. A 3-year-old child has episodes of sudden unsteadiness and vomiting with horizontal nystagmus.

'Best of five' questions

A 1.   C.

Premature thelarche is differentiated here from precocious puberty by the absence of pubic and axillary hair and the normal growth rate.

A 2.   C.

Erythema toxicum neonatorum is a common rash in well newborns occurring on the first 1–3 days of life. The pustules contain eosinophils. The rash subsides rapidly spontaneously.

Extended Matching Questions

A 1A.   D.

Cat scratch disease is due to a bacterial infection with *Bartonella henselae*. In around half of cases no history of scratch is obtained. In half of cases an inoculation papule or pustule is present which may last from days to months. Conjunctivitis and regional lymphadenopathy develop and there is mild malaise.

A 1B.   F.

Chicken pox infection is characterized by a fever and malaise, then the development of itchy papules and pustules initially post-auricular, the spreading to the neck, scalp, face, trunk and then the limbs. The lesions crust over, but all stages are seen at any one time as recurrent crops of vesicles appear.

A 2.   E.

This is most common in 1- to 3-year olds. It manifests with sudden onset of unsteadiness, vomiting and pallor. There is horizontal nystagmus and the child remains conscious. It is associated with ear infection.